KU-647-086

For Emma, Vicky and Brian (IFTB)

Contents

Acknowledgements

I would like to acknowledge the help of various colleagues in Manchester at the Polytechnic and at the Paterson Research Institute. In particular, a number of people who supplied information and/or photographs, including Diane Johnston, Ruth Abbott, Alan Curry, Micky Hoult, Chris Smith, Clair Cole and Mike Butler. Many thanks to Diane, Trudie and Ursula for much moral support in the 'dark days' and especially to my family, for whom the acronym 'WIFTB' (When I've finished the book) became all too familiar.

Introduction

Interleukins are proteins produced by leukocytes which function during inflammatory responses by acting on leukocytes or other targets (IUIS Nomenclature Committee, 1986). They behave as chemical mediators in immune responses, acting either as short-range messengers during interactions between cells or, like hormones, circulating in the blood and affecting cells at sites remote from their production. The term 'interleukin' was first used in 1979 and, in accord with current convention, an interleukin designation is now assigned to a protein which fits all the criteria only when the human gene for that product has been cloned and the amino acid sequence of the human protein determined. Seven molecules now have an interleukin designation. However, there are a number of very well-known proteins such as interferons, which fit all criteria for classification as interleukins, but which were named prior to the advent of the interleukin designation. Such molecules are interleukins in all but name and have been treated as such in this book.

Lymphokines are really interleukins which are produced by a particular type of leukocyte, namely, a lymphocyte, after appropriate stimulation in an immune response. Many lymphokines were named according to their biological activities in test systems and molecular characterization of these immunoregulatory molecules has, until the last few years, lagged well behind the detection of new activities.

The recent and enormous advances in our knowledge of lymphokines and interleukins is due to several major technological developments including the following:

(1) The ability to isolate single lymphocytes and grow them into clones of identical cells enables functional analysis of these cells and biochemical analysis of the mediators which they produce. The functional analysis of cells and their mediators has been greatly helped by the developments in monoclonal antibody technology, whereby relatively large amounts of homogeneous antibody can be produced in tissue culture.

(2) The techniques of recombinant DNA technology have enabled lymph-okines and interleukins to be produced in the quantities which are essential for biochemical and functional characterization of proteins. In addition, recombinant proteins are free from contamination with other, highly active factors which may be produced by stimulated leukocytes.

(3) Advances in biochemical preparative and analytical procedures have enabled DNA and proteins to be characterized more quickly and accurately using smaller amounts of precious material. In addition, the ability to store information about protein and DNA sequences in large databanks has greatly helped to identify similarities between different proteins. One effect of biochemical characterization has been to reduce the list of known lymphokines considerably since in many cases, different biological activities have been found to be the property of a single molecule.

There is a great deal of interest in these proteins because, while they provide an insight into the cellular interactions which takes place in immune responses, they can also be used as model systems for studying the processes of growth and differentiation in mammalian cells generally. Another, and major reason why these molecules are being studied so keenly is that, since they modulate immune responses, they have potential for use in medicine and, indeed, several are, or have been, the subject of clinical trials. Since the areas of medicine in which they might prove useful include cancer and immunodeficiency disease, there is also a good deal of commercial interest in these molecules.

In order to understand the importance of lymphokines and interleukins in the immune response and to appreciate their potential, Chapter 1 contains an overview of the immune responses which occur in higher vertebrates. Those readers who have already read the excellent textbooks in immunology referred to at the end of this chapter, will appreciate that this chapter can only be an outline of a very complex system. For those readers new to immunology, these books are recommended both personally and by many students who have discovered that immunology ranges far wider than microbial serology and immunodiffusion tests. Chapters 2 and 3 are concerned with methodology in lymphokine research including how they are produced, characterized and assayed. Chapters 4 to 10 cover particular molecules which have been chosen either because they are central to the immune response, the subject of intense research activity, or have real or potential clinical and commercial interest (and frequently all three). However, as the reader will discover, interleukins rarely work in isolation; synergisms occur between different molecules and several interleukins have overlapping activities. The final chapter attempts to summarize these overlapping functions and to anticipate the future directions of research into these fascinating molecules.

The Immune Response

Introduction

The immune system is a complex network of cells and macromolecules which interact to eliminate disease-producing (pathogenic) microorganisms from the body. Individuals whose immune systems have failed to develop properly, or whose immunity has been compromised by infection with the human immunodeficiency virus (HIV) suffer life-threatening infections of bacterial, viral, fungal, protozoal or helminthic origin. However, the immune system does not only eliminate pathogens and similar immune responses are shown towards all manner of microorganisms as well as macromolecules such as proteins and glycoproteins which are all removed by similar mechanisms. A limited form of immune response is even shown towards inert particles, as can be seen, for example, when a splinter of wood is left under the skin for several days. The immune system can therefore be said to have a dual function, namely to distinguish that which is 'self' from that which is not, and secondly, to eliminate 'non-self'.

Non-specific and specific immune systems

The components of the immune system can be put into one of two categories according to the specificity of their action. Some cells and macromolecules are completely non-specific and will act on any 'non-self' components which enter the body. Others are completely specific for a particular microorganism or protein and only react to that 'foreign' component. In general, non-specific mechanisms form the first arm of the defence against microorganisms whereas specific immunity takes some time to develop after exposure to a microorganism. For this reason, non-specific immunity is often said to be innate (inborn), whereas specific immunity is 'acquired' during the course of an infection. The division of the immune system into these two groups can be misleading if it is not emphasized that the two systems interact at all stages of the response. So, for example, cells without specificity can stimulate specific cells and specific cells, when stimulated, secrete products which heighten the activity of non-specific cells.

NON-SPECIFIC DEFENCE

All animals have barriers which prevent the entry of microorganisms. The most obvious barrier is the skin but mucosal surfaces which line the gastrointestinal, respiratory and genitourinary tracts represent large surface areas separating the 'outside' from the 'inside' of the body. These mucosal surfaces are protected by chemicals (such as HCl in the stomach), by proteins such as mucus, which prevents bacteria from adhering to the membrane itself, and enzymes such as lysozyme, which dissolves the cell walls of bacteria. Once these barriers are breached, other non-specific proteins and cells can limit the spread of the infection. Proteins such as interferon (IFN) and complement provide non-specific defences against viruses and bacteria, respectively.

Interferons are proteins which protect cells from viral infection by inducing the synthesis of molecules which interfere with viral replication. Classically, interferons are produced by virus infected cells and belong to one of two classes, known as interferons α and β. There is, however, a third class, IFN-γ, which differs both structurally and functionally from these and is the product of a specific immune response.

Complement is the collective name for a group of proteins found in plasma and intercellular fluids which can lyse bacteria and promote their phagocytosis by white blood cells. Complement proteins work sequentially, the sequence being triggered (or activated) by bacterial cell-wall components or by antibodies (specific protein products of a specific immune response). Activation of complement by antibodies or bacterial cell walls utilizes different complement proteins but has similar end results.

Non-specific cells of the immune system

Phagocytic cells form an important arm of the non-specific defences against pathogens. Microorganisms taken up by phagocytes are destroyed by one of several mechanisms. Lysosomes may fuse with the phagocytic vacuole and discharge hydrolytic enzymes onto the organism. At the same time, a burst of aerobic respiration which accompanies phagocytosis can result in the production of oxygen metabolites such as superoxide and hydrogen peroxide which have bactericidal properties. Two types of phagocytic cell are found in the body: the polymorphonuclear leukocyte (PMN) and the monocyte.

Polymorphonuclear leukocytes.   PMN constitute the predominant type of white cell in the blood. Three types exist but the most abundant, and the only one with significant phagocytic activity is the neutrophilic PMN *(neutrophil)* which makes up approximately 60% of blood leukocytes. The neutrophil is 12–15 μm in diameter and has a characteristic multi-lobed nucleus and granular cytoplasm (Fig. 1.1). Neutrophils, like all leukocytes, enter the circulation from their site of production in the bone marrow. They are short-lived cells which are continually and steadily replaced from the bone marrow. During an infection, however, the numbers of circulating neutrophils can increase dramatically and this is influenced by several interleukins including IL-1 and IL-6.

Neutrophils are important in inflammation, a series of events which takes place at the site of any tissue damage. Chemical mediators released from damaged tissues cause dilation of blood vessels (Fig. 1.2) which results in increased blood flow and reddening of the area. The endothelial cells which line the blood vessels move apart and neutrophils, which adhere to the endothelial cells, migrate between the endothelial cells and across the basement membrane, and accumulate at the site of injury. At the same time the vessels become more permeable to plasma which also accumulates in the area bringing with it complement proteins and antibodies built up from previous immune reactions. This inflammatory response occurs at the site of any tissue damage or infection. For example, at a site of chronic tissue damage such as might occur if a splinter of wood were left in the skin, neutrophils continue to build up at the site forming an 'inflammatory exudate'. This accumulation of cells and fluid forms the character- istic pus in an area of infection. Neutrophils can also be attracted chemotactically to sites of infection by activated complement proteins.

Monocytes.   Monocytes account for approximately 5% of total blood leuko- cytes. They have a rounded nucleus which is characteristically indented, and abundant cytoplasm. The blood monocyte represents a half-way stage in the development of this phagocytic cell. Produced in the bone marrow, monocytes circulate in the blood, sometimes for weeks, then enter other tissues and develop into tissue macrophages which are larger cells, with greater phagocytic capability (Fig. 1.1). The activity of macrophages can be greatly increased by products of the specific immune response and, in particular, the lymphokine IFN-γ. Macrophages are found in almost all tissues (see Table 1.1) but are especially abundant in those organs which make up the *reticuloendothelial system* (RES) the function of which is to filter out foreign material from the blood and tissues. The phagocytosis of microorganisms, especially Gram-negative bacteria or bacterial endotoxins, by monocytes and macrophages results in the release from these cells of IL-1, IL-6 and tumour necrosis factor (TNF) which are important in stimulating both specific and non-specific responses.

In addition to the phagocytic cells, other blood leukocytes are involved in different aspects of non-specific immunity. Amongst these are two other types of PMN: eosinophils and basophils, and the large granular lymphocytes (LGL) (see Fig. 1.1).

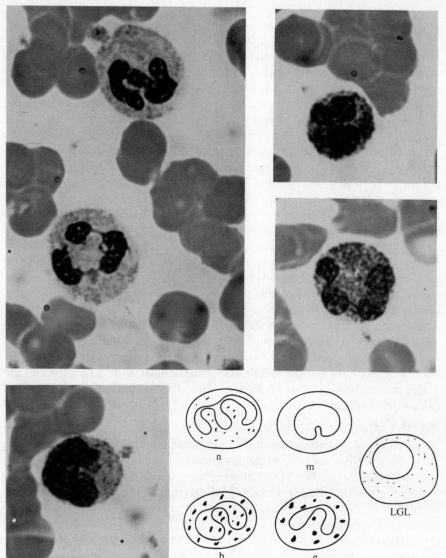

Fig. 1.1 Cells of the non-specific immune system. The different leukocytes in the blood can be distinguished after differential staining with a combination of Jenner and Giemsa stains (×630). The *neutrophil* (n) has a pale granular cytoplasm and a multilobed nucleus. It is the most abundant leukocyte in the blood and is phagocytic. *Monocytes* (m) comprise 5% of leukocytes. They have a 'horseshoe' nucleus and pale cytoplasm. In the tissues they develop into macrophages. The *eosinophil* (e) has prominent pink-staining cytoplasmic granules and a bilobed nucleus. It constitutes about 2% of leukocytes in health but can increase considerably (a condition known as eosinophilia) in patients with parasitic infection. The *basophil* (b) has blue-staining cytoplasmic granules containing pharmacological mediators such as histamine. The basophil develops into a mast cell in the tissues. *Large granular lymphocytes* (LGL) have rounded nuclei and less prominent cytoplasmic granules. Some have natural killer activity and spontaneously destroy tumour cells and virus-infected cells.

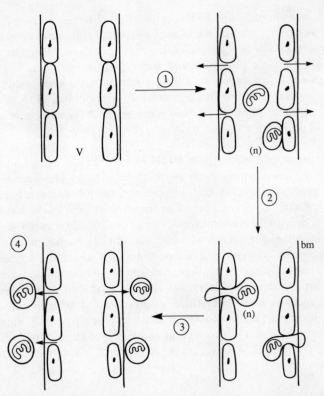

Fig. 1.2 Neutrophils and inflammation. The blood vessel (v) is lined with endothelial cells which are closely apposed. In inflammation, histamine from mast cells dilates blood vessels, making them more permeable to plasma. The endothelial cells move apart, creating intercellular gaps (1). Neutrophils (n) adhere to the endothelial cells (2) and move between the endothelial cells (3) and across the basement membrane (bm). The neutrophils accumulate at the inflammatory site (4) and may also be attracted there by some complement proteins.

Table 1.1 Distribution of monocytes/macrophages

Tissue	Name
Blood*	Monocyte
Spleen*	Macrophages
Lymph nodes*	Macrophages
Lungs*	Alveolar macrophages
Liver*	Kupffer cells
Brain	Microglia
Bone	Osteoclasts
Renal glomeruli	Mesangial cells
Peritoneum	Peritoneal macrophages

*Tissues forming part of the reticuloendothelial system.

Eosinophil.   Eosinophils are PMNs with bilobed nuclei and very prominent granules which take up acidic stains such as eosin. Eosinophils constitute a very minor proportion of leukocytes (usually <2%) but the numbers are elevated in patients with parasitic infections and some allergies including hay fever and allergic asthma. Eosinophils can kill parasitic worms *in vitro*, especially if the worms are coated with specific antibody. A lymphokine, IL-5, which is the product of a specific immune response, increases both the number of eosinophils in the blood and their cytotoxicity.

Basophils.   Basophils are a type of PMN with prominent cytoplasmic granules which take up basic stains such as methylene blue. The granules contain numerous pharmacologically active agents including histamine, heparin and a chemotactic factor for eosinophils. The tissue equivalent of the basophil is the mast cell which is found predominantly in mucosal membranes of the respiratory and gastrointestinal surfaces as well as in the skin. In particular circumstances, perhaps as a result of tissue damage or often as a result of a specific immune response to parasitic infections, these mediators are released and can stimulate inflammation by dilating blood vessels and attracting eosinophils. Some mediators, such as histamine, cause contraction of smooth muscle. When released by local mast cells, these mediators may play a role in the elimination of parasites from the gut. The production and differentiation of mast cells can be modified by IL-3 and IL-4 which are the products of cells of the specific immune response.

Large granular lymphocytes (LGL).   Approximately 5–10% of blood leuko-cytes are LGL (see Fig 1.1). These are cells with rounded nuclei, and abundant granular cytoplasm. LGL are cytotoxic cells with two types of cytotoxic activity: some LGL spontaneously kill a restricted range of cultured tumour cells, and virus-infected cells, and are known as *natural killer (NK)* cells. In addition, some LGL can kill antibody-coated target cells, an activity which is known as *antibody-dependent cellular cytotoxicity (ADCC)*. NK and ADCC activities are probably carried out by overlapping populations, the majority of LGL carrying out both activities. The cytotoxic capacity of LGL is increased by lymphokines such as IL-2 and IFN-γ.

THE SPECIFIC IMMUNE RESPONSE

When an individual is infected for the first time with a pathogen such as rubella (German measles), non-specific immune mechanisms are often insufficient to stop the pathogen from replicating, spreading and causing disease. Individuals recover from infections with rubella or other pathogens because, during the course of the infection, cells with specificity for the virus proliferate and develop into effector cells. Depending on the type of cell stimulated, these effector cells either produce specific proteins (antibodies) which bind to the virus, triggering its

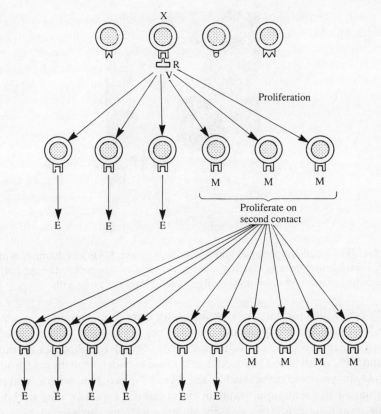

Fig. 1.3 The specific immune response. The cell X is specific for a virus (V) because it has cell-surface receptors for that virus. Contact with the virus causes only cells X to proliferate, producing a clone of cells with identical specificity. Some of these cells develop into effector cells (E) which deal with the virus while other cells remain as memory cells (M) which can respond on the second contact with the immunogen. Because there are more cells with the 'right' receptor, the response is better than before.

elimination, or they become cytotoxic cells, endowed with the capacity to kill the cells that are infected with the virus. Some of the progeny of the stimulated cell do not complete differentiation but remain as 'memory' cells, increasing the population of cells with specificity for the virus so that, on second exposure, an immune response is detected more rapidly (Fig. 1.3). Individuals who recover from an infection are therefore said to be 'immune' to that infectious agent. When next exposed to the same agent, they not only have antibodies and/or cytotoxic cells from the previous exposure, but a much more rapid response results in elimination of the infectious agent often before clinical symptoms develop.

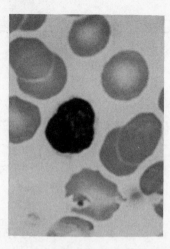

Fig. 1.4 The small lymphocyte. Small lymphocytes are 7–9 μm in diameter with a large, rounded and densely staining nucleus. At least two populations exist but these are indistinguishable in a conventionally stained blood smear ($\times$ 630).

The cells which produce the specific response are small lymphocytes which are found in the blood and lymphoid tissues. They are the only cells in the immune system which are endowed with specificity. Small lymphocytes account for around 25% of all blood leukocytes and are also widely distributed throughout the body in lymphoid tissues such as the thymus, spleen, lymph nodes and tonsils. They have a distinctive appearance in blood smears. Typically, they are 7–9 μm in diameter and have a large, densely staining nucleus surrounded by a rim of cytoplasm (Fig. 1.4). At the ultrastructural level, there are very few organelles and little endoplasmic reticulum.

Immunogens, antigens and epitopes

The specific immune response is not shown towards all 'non-self' components. For example, antibodies are not produced against wood splinters or carbon particles in tobacco smoke. The term *immunogen* (previously *antigen*), is used to describe a cell, or macromolecule which induces a specific immune response. The term 'antigen' is sometimes limited to a molecule which combines with the products of the immune response but which by itself may not necessarily stimulate an immune response.

The ability of an immunogen to stimulate a specific immune response depends on several factors including the size of the molecule, the degree of internal variety in the structure and the degree of 'foreignness'. While there are no hard and fast rules, the smallest naturally occurring protein which is immunogenic is probably insulin, which has a molecular weight of 5 kilodaltons (5 kDa). Proteins, which have great internal variety, being composed of over 20 different amino acids

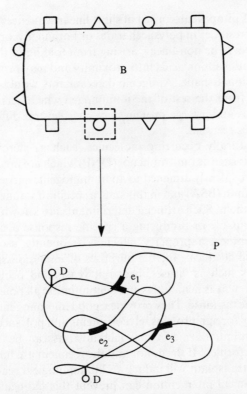

Fig. 1.5 Immunogens, epitopes and haptens. A bacterium (B) is an immunogen which can be likened to a 'package' of proteins and glycoproteins, each of which could be immunogenic on its own. A membrane protein (P) contains regions to which the cells of the specific immune system respond. These are known as 'epitopes' and are not immunogenic in isolation. A single protein may have several different epitopes e_1, e_2 and e_3 for example, each of which stimulates a specific cell. Small synthetic groups, such as dinitrophenol (D), which are not immunogenic, can be covalently attached to a protein where they stimulate a specific immune response. In such cases these small molecules are known as 'haptens'.

present in sequences characteristic of an individual protein, are more immunogenic than polysaccharides which comprise relatively few different monosaccharide residues. At the same time, the immunogenicity of a protein will depend on the evolutionary relationship between that protein and the animal exposed to it. For example, human proteins are more immunogenic in mice than in primates where the evolutionary relationship is closer.

All small lymphocytes have cell-surface receptors which are specific, not for the whole immunogen, but for small regions of the molecule known as 'antigenic determinants' or *epitopes* (Fig. 1.5). Similarly, the cytotoxic cells and antibodies produced during the immune response are specific for the epitopes which induced their production. Epitopes can consist of short linear sequences of amino acids in proteins, glycosyl residues in polysaccharides or both in glycoproteins. Alternatively, an epitope may be non-linear, arising from folding of the protein, which brings non-sequential amino acids into proximity and may produce a characteristic three-dimensional shape. Antigenic determinants would not be immunogenic in isolation from the rest of the immunogen which acts as a 'carrier' for individual epitopes and a large protein may have several different epitopes to which lymphocytes respond.

Many small naturally occurring molecules, such as steroid hormones, or synthetic chemicals such as dinitrophenol (DNP) which are not immunogenic on their own can be covalently attached to an immunogenic carrier protein such as bovine serum albumin (BSA) and in this state a specific immune response may be produced against them. Such artificial determinants are known as *haptens*. Thus an individual is capable of producing a specific response against a seemingly endless list of haptens, a property which is frequently used when making antibodies to small chemicals for the purposes of immunoassay.

Microorganisms such as viruses, bacteria, yeasts and protozoa and multicellular organisms such as nematodes and helminths are all potent stimulators of the specific immune response. They provide a good immunogenic stimulus, being 'packages' of many foreign proteins, glycoproteins and polysaccharides. Indeed, any cells can be immunogenic in the right host, as can be seen when tissue transplants are performed. If the donor and the recipient are not identical twins, the immunogenic transplant will induce an immunological reaction against the graft, although clinical intervention can prevent this happening. Even cancer cells arising within an individual can be immunogenic and cytotoxic cells and antibodies may be produced against the tumour cells, although in most spontaneously arising tumours this host response is usually weak.

Role of small lymphocytes in specific immunity

All small lymphocytes are derived ultimately from the bone marrow but different patterns of development separate them into two major populations with differing functions. These two populations are known as *T-* and *B-lymphocytes* according to whether part of their development takes place in the thymus (T = thymus dependent). When B-lymphocytes are stimulated with specific immunogens they proliferate and develop into antibody-secreting cells called 'plasma cells', a process which is known as *humoral immunity*. The antibodies which are secreted are specific glycoproteins which bind to an epitope and stimulate destruction of the immunogen, by phagocytic cells and LGL. There are at least two functionally distinct populations of T-lymphocytes, one of which (Tc) is responsible for *cell-mediated immunity*, in which specific T-cells are stimulated to proliferate and develop into cytotoxic T-lymphocytes (CTL) which can kill cells infected with a virus against which they were induced. Antigen-induced proliferation and differentiation of both CTL and plasma cells, is dependent on the presence of

Table 1.2 Some useful cell differentiation antigens on human leukocytes

Differentiation antigen*	Distribution	Representative monoclonal antibody**
CD3	Mature T-cells	OKT3
CD4	Helper T-cells (65% of peripheral T-cells)	OKT4
CD8	Cytotoxic/suppressor T-cells (35% of peripheral T-cells)	OKT8
CD14	Monocytes	Mo 2
CD16	Granulocytes, NK cells	Leu 11
CD19	B-cells	B4

* The CD classification refers to a 'cluster of determinants' which were recognized by a range of different monoclonal antibodies. International workshops showed that all the antibodies assigned to one group were detecting the same protein although not necessarily the same epitope on that protein. Thus, CD does not strictly mean 'cell differentiation'.
** These monoclonal antibodies are all mouse immunoglobulins. If they are incubated with cells expressing the determinant, they bind to that cell and can be visualized by incubating the cell with a labelled antibody to mouse immunoglobulin. Suitable labels include a fluorescent marker such as fluorescein isothiocyanate, which produces an apple green fluorescence when the cells are irradiated with ultraviolet light, or an enzyme such as horseradish peroxidase which produces a coloured product when incubated with an appropriate substrate.

stimulatory factors which are produced by another type of T-lymphocyte known as a helper T-cell (T_H). B- and T-lymphocytes are morphologically identical at the level of the light microscopic although they can be distinguished by their characteristic cell-surface proteins. Table 1.2 shows some useful surface markers which can be used to distinguish different populations of leukocytes.

Development of T-lymphocytes

The mammalian tissues which are concerned with the development of lymphocytes are the fetal liver, bone marrow and the thymus. In birds there is, in addition to the thymus, another lymphoid organ associated with the hind-gut and known as the bursa of Fabricius. The fetal liver, and later the bone marrow, contain stem cells which, by repeated division, give rise to cells capable of developing into any of the white cells in the blood. During embryonic development, some lymphocyte precursors leave the bone marrow and enter the thymus, a lympho-epithelial organ situated centrally in the upper anterior chest. In the thymus, lymphocyte precursors undergo a period of development generally known as 'thymic processing', during which period the cells both acquire cell-surface receptors which endow them with specificity for foreign

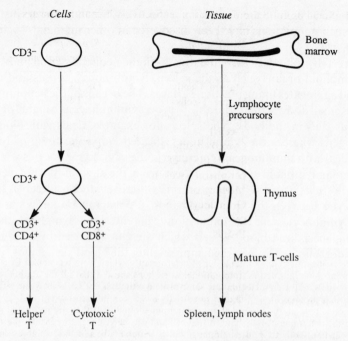

Fig. 1.6 Development of T-lymphocytes. Stem cells in the bone marrow give rise to lymphocyte precursors which leave the bone marrow in embryonic life and seed the thymus. In the thymus they develop into mature T-cells, characterized by specific antigen receptors and the presence of the CD3 protein. Mature T-cells which leave the thymus belong to one of two populations: helper T-cells, which also have the CD4 membrane glycoprotein, and cytotoxic T-cells which are positive for CD8. The mature T-cells travel to the secondary lymphoid tissues such as the spleen and lymph nodes and recirculate between the blood and these lymphoid tissues.

proteins, microorganisms, etc. and they also become committed to a particular function (Fig. 1.6).

The development of T-lymphocytes during this period of processing can be followed to some extent by looking at the acquisition of certain cell-surface proteins which can act as markers of differentiation. As thymic lymphocytes mature they both lose and acquire cell differentiation antigens. These antigens are integral membrane glycoproteins. For example, during development in the thymus, maturing T-cells start to express CD3, a protein which is permanently expressed on mature T-lymphocytes. Some time after acquisition of the CD3 marker, thymic lymphocytes separate into two distinct populations which then leave the thymus and 'seed' the lymphoid tissues distributed throughout the body. These two populations can be distinguished because one population expresses both the CD3 marker and another glycoprotein called CD4 whereas the second population expresses both CD3 and CD8. The majority of T-cells expressing CD4 or CD8 are T_H and T_C, respectively. Similar markers distinguishing two such populations have been discovered in other mammals such as mice and rats.

Mature T-lymphocytes leave the thymus in the neonatal period and 'seed' the other lymphoid organs such as the spleen, lymph nodes, tonsils and the local lymphoid aggregates lining mucosal surfaces. The organs of the lymphoid system are widespread and are therefore able to process immunogens capable of entering at various sites in the body. The spleen, for example, deals with blood-borne immunogens whereas the lymph nodes, located along the route of lymphatic vessels, deal with immunogens, entering via the skin. Lymphocytes which settle in particular lymphoid tissues after exit from the thymus do not necessarily remain in that tissue. On the contrary, there is a considerable traffic of lymphocytes between the blood and lymph, a phenomenon known as *recirculation*. Lymphocytes in the circulation can enter the lymphoid tissues by traversing specialized blood vessels which are characterized by a columnar or 'high' endothelium. Those in the lymph re-enter the blood via a major lymphatic vessel, the right thoracic duct. Since individual lymphocytes are specific for a single epitope, the recirculation of small lymphocytes makes the likelihood greater that an individual lymphocyte will meet the appropriate epitope if an immunogen gains entry to the body. Consequently, the number of lymphocytes specific for an individual epitope is less than would be necessary if all lymphoid tissues had a full complement of specific, but static, cells.

Functions of T-lymphocytes. The effects of neonatal thymectomy in mice have been well-known for at least twenty years. Such animals have no cell-mediated immunity, they suffer viral infections, and are unable to reject grafts of foreign skin, indicating that T-lymphocytes are essential for these activities. In immunocompetent animals, recognition of viral epitopes by specific CD8$^+$ T-lymphocytes leads to proliferation and differentiation of these cells into cytotoxic T-lymphocytes (CTL) (Fig. 1.7) which can kill, specifically, virus-infected cells and in doing so prevent viral replication. The destruction of virus-infected cells by specific CTL is thought to be mediated by short-range toxins released by the CTL following binding to the specific epitope. In addition to direct cytotoxicity, CD8$^+$ cells produce some lymphokines including IFN-γ, IL-2 and tumour necrosis factor β (TNF-β). All three molecules modulate a range of immunological activities. Some CD8$^+$ cells can also suppress immune responses, for example, to 'self' antigens. It is not clear whether these 'suppressor' cells represent a different or overlapping population or indeed whether they represent the same population at different developmental stages.

The majority of T-cells which express the CD4 membrane protein are helper T-lymphocytes (T_H). When these cells are stimulated during an immune response they produce a range of lymphokines, including growth and differentiation factors for CD8$^+$ and B-lymphocytes, and factors which stimulate the activities of a wide range of cells including macrophages, NK cells and bone-marrow stem

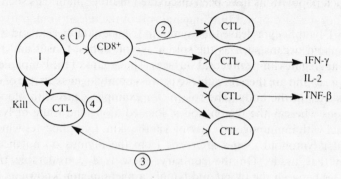

(a) Development of cytotoxic T-lymphocyte

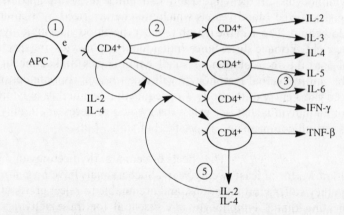

(b) Development of 'immune' Helper T-cells

Fig. 1.7 Immunity in T-lymphocytes. (a) Cytotoxic T-lymphocytes. (1) T-lymphocytes bearing the CD8 glycoprotein (Tc) respond to a foreign epitope (e) by proliferation and differentiation (2) to form a clone of cytotoxic T-lymphocytes (CTL) with specificity for the same epitope. CTL bind to the epitope and destroy the immunogen extracellularly (3,4). CTL also produce some lymphokines including IFN-γ, IL-2 and TNF-β. Development of CTL requires lymphokines from stimulated helper T-cells.
(b) Helper T-cells. (1) T-lymphocytes positive for CD4 respond to epitopes 'presented' to them by antigen-presenting cells (APC). Stimulated T_H proliferate (2) and produce a range of lymphokines (3) some of which (IL-2 and IL-4) support proliferation of both CD4$^+$ (4) and CD8$^+$ cells.

cells (see Fig. 1.7). T_H are central to a specific immune response and their depletion, as for example in AIDS, can result in much increased susceptibility to infection. The normal ratio of CD4$^+$:CD8$^+$ cells in the blood of healthy individuals is 2:1 but as a consequence of infection with the human immunodeficiency virus (HIV) which infects and destroys cells expressing the CD4 molecule, the ratio can be as low as 0.5: 1.0 with the result that these patients are prone to a wide range of opportunistic pathogens.

T-lymphocytes also play a fundamental role in the rejection of grafts but the precise roles of T_H and T_C in this phenomenon are still being evaluated. $CD8^+$ cells removed from an animal undergoing graft rejection have been shown to destroy cells of the graft *in vitro*. On the other hand, $CD4^+$ cells may contribute to graft destruction by, for example, providing growth factors for cytotoxic cells, and by producing lymphokines which recruit other cytotoxic cells, such as macrophages, or which render the graft more susceptible to killing.

Recognition of antigen by T-lymphocytes. The recognition of specific epitopes by T-lymphocytes is a very complex phenomenon, because it depends, not only on the presence of specific T-cell receptors, but also on the recognition, at the same time, of certain 'self' antigens. These 'self' antigens are cell-surface proteins which are encoded by genes found within a region of the genome known as the *major histocompatibility complex* (MHC). Moreover, the situation is complicated by the fact that $CD4^+$ and $CD8^+$ T-lymphocytes recognize different 'self' antigens, encoded by different regions of the MHC. In addition, $CD4^+$ cells only respond to antigen when it is presented to them, in association with MHC antigens, by specialized antigen-presenting cells. In order, therefore, to understand the complexities of these interactions, an explanation is needed of the nature of T-cell receptors, of the MHC and its products, and of antigen-presenting cells.

The T-cell receptor. All T-lymphocytes have specific receptors for an individual epitope. Each receptor is unique in terms of amino acid sequence although the overall secondary and tertiary structures of T-cell receptors are the same in all T-lymphocytes. The receptor, Ti (Fig. 1.8) consists of two non-identical polypeptide chains: an α-chain with a molecular weight of 43 kDa and a β-chain with a molecular weight of 40 kDa. Both chains have variable (V) regions in which the amino acid sequence determines the epitope specificity. These V regions are located at the amino terminal end of the molecule. The carboxy-terminal ends have fairly constant (C) amino acid sequences. The V and C regions of the T-cell receptor are the products of different genes which are joined together during development of the cell. An immature T-lymphocyte is potentially capable of producing a T-cell receptor of any specificity but during development a process of gene rearrangements and gene deletions means that a mature T-lymphocyte is confined to producing a receptor of a single specificity. The T-cell receptor is always found in a complex with another, invariant, molecule which in humans is the CD3 protein, present on all mature T-cells. CD3 is a complex of at least three different polypeptide chains which, in combination with Ti, forms the T-cell receptor complex. Whereas the role of the variant Ti is to bind antigen, T3 appears to act as a transducing protein, transmitting the activation signal across the cell membrane to reactive molecules in the cytoplasm.

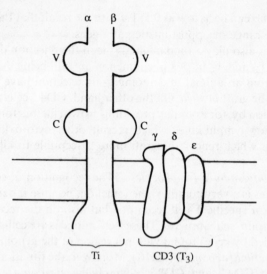

Fig. 1.8 The T-cell receptor complex. The specific receptor on T-cells is Ti, a dimer made up of two non-identical polypeptide chains, α and β, with variable (V) and constant (C) regions. The specific receptor is always associated with the CD3 protein which is invariant. CD3 is composed of at least three polypeptide chains (γ, δ and ε) and is concerned with the transmission of signals across the membrane once Ti has bound specific epitope.

The major histocompatibility complex (MHC)

The MHC is a region of the genome which encodes integral membrane glycoproteins of fundamental importance in the regulation of the immune response and the ability to distinguish 'self' and 'non-self'. The discovery of the MHC was the result of pioneering work during the 1930s and 1940s in the fields of transplantation and tumour immunology. In laboratory experiments with mice the rejection of grafts was related to differences in cell-surface 'histocompatibility' antigens, mapping to the H2 region, on chromosome 17, which is the mouse MHC. Similar regions have been found in all the mammalian species so far studied, the human equivalent being the HLA system located on chromosome 6.

The immunological significance of the MHC was not fully appreciated until 1973 when the phenomenon of MHC restriction was first observed. In this instance, virus-specific CTL were only able to kill virus-infected cells *in vitro* if the target cells expressed the same MHC determinants as the CTL. This phenomenon was the first demonstration that immune interactions are restricted to cells expressing recognizable, i.e. self, MHC determinants.

The MHC region of man and the mouse (Fig. 1.9) encodes three groups of genes known as Class I, II and III. Class I genes code for those determinants

(a) HLA of man

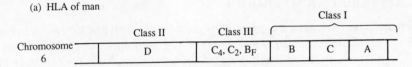

(b) H2 of mouse

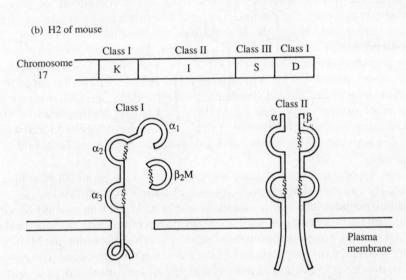

Fig. 1.9 The major histocompatibility complex of man and mouse. The MHC of man (HLA) and mouse (H2) is located on chromosome 6 and 17, respectively. In man, Class I proteins are coded by genes in the A, B and C regions. Class II are encoded within the D region, at three sub-loci: DP, DQ and DR. Class III genes specify some complement proteins. In the H2 complex, the K and D regions code for Class I proteins and the I region the Class II. The S region also encodes some complement proteins. Class I proteins consist of an α-chain of 45 kDa and β_2-microglobulin (12 kDa). Class II proteins consist of two polypeptide chains: α (34 kDa) and β (28 kDa) held together by non-covalent binding.

which restrict the activity of cytotoxic T-cells. These molecules are also the transplantation antigens, i.e. they induce graft rejection. The products of Class II genes act as restriction elements for the interaction of antigen-presenting cells with helper T-cells while Class III genes encode some complement proteins. Recently, some lymphokine genes have also been located within the MHC which is interesting mainly because some lymphokines also regulate the expression of MHC proteins. In the mouse, differences in the ability to respond to a particular antigen have been traced to differences in the I region leading to the proposal that this region contains immune response (Ir) genes. The human equivalent of the I region is HLA-D, which is further subdivided into three sub-loci: DP, DQ and DR.

CLASS I GENES AND PRODUCTS

Human Class I antigens are encoded by genes in the A, B and C regions in man. All the genetic loci are polyallelic, that is, they exist in many alternative forms in the population, an individual having two genes at the A locus (one on each of a pair of homologous chromosomes), two B genes and two C genes. These allelic genes present on homologous chromosomes are co-dominant so that an individual possessing, for example, the gene A3 (an allele at the A locus of one chromosome) and A5 on the homologous chromosome will have both the protein products expressed in the cell membrane. The extreme polymorphism of these genes makes it highly unlikely that any two unrelated individuals possess an identical complement of HLA antigens on their cell membranes but, since these genes are inherited in a Mendelian fashion and recombination events are rare, the chances of siblings possessing HLA identity or partial identity are of course much higher. Similarly, highly inbred strains of mice have been produced where all individuals express identical Class I gene products. Such animals are said to be syngeneic.

Class I proteins are found on all nucleated cells and all have a similar secondary structure. Each protein consists of a single transmembrane glycosylated polypeptide chain with a molecular weight of 45 000 (the α-chain) which is always found in association with a smaller polypeptide chain of 12 000 called $\beta_2 M$ which does not cross the cell membrane, is not encoded within the MHC but which is essential for the expression of the α-chain in the membrane. The α-chain can be divided into three extracellular regions, or domains called α_1, α_2 and α_3. The allelic variation in the products of different A, B and C genes is found most commonly in the α_1 and α_2 domains.

CLASS II GENES AND PRODUCTS

Class II genes are located in the I region of the H2 complex in mice and in the D region of the human HLA region. Moreover, the D region contains three sub-loci namely DP, DQ and DR. Class II gene products are restricted to a few cell types including monocytes, macrophages, B-cells, thymus epithelium and activated, but not resting, T-cells. The Class II products on thymic epithelium are important in the development of the immune response because mature T-cells only recognize those molecules which were expressed in the thymus during the vital period of thymic processing. In addition, some cells, such as those of endothelium, can be induced to express Class II molecules if treated with lymphokines such as IFN-γ and TNF, and this may have implications for the development of autoimmune disease. Class II products are heterodimers consisting of an α-chain of 30–34 kDa and a β-chain of 26–29 kDa both of which are transmembrane. The extracellular portion of both chains contains two domains and allelic variation occurs almost entirely in the β-chain.

ANTIGEN-PRESENTING CELLS (APC) AND CLASS II PROTEINS

The majority of immunogens fail to stimulate helper T-lymphocytes unless they are presented to them by APC. The importance of APC was first discovered during attempts to stimulate antibody production *in vitro* when it was shown that antibody was produced only if monocytes or macrophages were present in the cultures. In addition, antibody production could be initiated *in vitro* in the absence of any 'free' immunogen by exposing lymphocytes to macrophages which have been incubated with immunogen for approximately 60 min. Macrophages which had been fixed in formaldehyde prior to incubation with antigen were unable to stimulate lymphocytes *in vitro*, indicating that their role is more than that of passively absorbing antigen onto their surface. Antigen-presenting cells (APC) such as the macrophage are essential for the initiation of CMI as well as humoral immunity. For example, T-lymphocytes from an immunized animal will proliferate *in vitro* if exposed to that antigen as long as APC are also present.

Several features are essential for a cell to present antigen. First, the antigen is taken into the cell where it is 'processed'. Processing appears to involve metabolic steps during which the antigen is broken down, in acidic intracellular compartments distinct from the lysosomes. The smaller fragments are then inserted into the membrane of the APC in such a way that they associate with Class II molecules of the MHC (Fig. 1.10). It is the complex of antigen with Class II molecules which is thought to be recognized by the antigen-specific T_H. For some polypeptide antigens, the processing event may involve a denaturation rather than proteolytic cleavage. The effect of denaturation may simply be to uncover that part of the molecule capable of associating with Class II determinants. Finally, the APC also produces IL-1 which stimulates the helper T-cell.

Several cell types are capable of presenting antigen to the helper T-cell and these are shown in Table 1.3. Although monocytes and macrophages do act as APC, the dendritic cells which are a frequent, although minor contaminant of

Table 1.3 Antigen presenting cells and their location

Cell type	Location
Monocytes	Blood
Macrophages	Reticuloendothelial tissues
B-lymphocytes	Blood and lymphoid tissues
Dendritic cells	Blood
Langerhans cell	Skin
Interdigitating cell	Lymph node
Veiled cell	Efferent lymph (i.e. lymph draining from a lymph node)

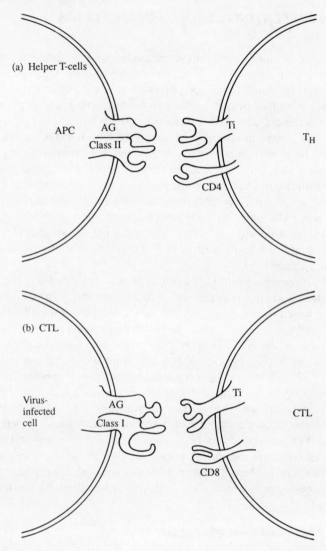

Fig. 1.10   Interaction between the T-cell receptor and antigen. (a) Helper T-cells.
The antigen-presenting cell (APC) processes antigen internally, then re-expresses it on
the cell membrane complexed with Class II molecules. The T-cell receptor, Ti,
recognizes the epitope and the variant regions of the Class II molecule. In addition
(though not represented here) the binding is strengthened by interaction between the
CD4 protein and the invariant regions of the Class II.
(b) Cytotoxic T-cells. CTL recognize antigen (AG) such as viral protein, on the
surface of a virus-infected cell. CTL also recognize the variant regions of the Class I
molecules. In addition, binding may be strengthened by interaction between the CD8
molecule and the invariant region of the Class I.

this population, are much more efficient at antigen presentation and may have a more significant APC function *in vivo*. Langerhans cells in the skin process and present immunogens which have entered through the skin. These cells travel to the draining lymph node where they present antigen to T-cells in the deep cortex. Many of the cells listed have multiple membrane processes resulting in a relatively large surface area for antigen presentation. B-lymphocytes, which also express Class II molecules can also present antigen to helper T-cells and, indeed, a physical interaction between T- and B-lymphocytes seems to be necessary in order to achieve activation, proliferation and differentiation of B-lymphocytes in humoral immunity.

INTERACTION OF T-CELLS AND APC

The recognition of antigen on the surface of antigen-presenting cells is a complex process involving Ti, and the CD4 molecule of the helper T-cell and Class II molecules on the APC. The nature of this recognition is the subject of much intense research activity and a complete understanding of the interaction of these molecules is dependent on greater knowledge of their tertiary structures. The primary amino acid sequences of Class II molecules have been known for some time but the three-dimensional structure of one such molecule has only recently been proposed.

The T_H cell responds to antigen presented on the surface of APC in conjunction with MHC Class II proteins and IL-1 made by the latter. It is likely that the T-cell receptor (Ti) recognizes the antigen in association with the polymorphic (i.e. variant) regions of the Class II molecules (see Fig. 1.10). The CD4 molecule on the surface of T_H may also be involved in the recognition process but in a non-specific manner. CD4 is invariant and is thought to bind to the non-polymorphic regions of the Class II molecules where its role may be to strengthen the interaction between the two cells so that activation of the helper T-cell can occur. Successful recognition of antigen in this manner by a specific T_H together with the second signal delivered by IL-1 initiates the release of lymphokines from T_H. The release of lymphokines from helper T-cells is sequential. It seems likely that IL-2 is released first and that this then stimulates the producer cell in an autocrine manner to release a range of lymphokines including IL-2, IL-3, IL-4, IL-5, IL-6, IFN-γ and TNF-β. In mice, there is evidence for the existence of at least two populations of helper T-cells with different patterns of lymphokine production.

RECOGNITION OF ANTIGEN BY CD8$^+$ CELLS

T-lymphocytes bearing the CD8 molecule recognize antigen on the surface of virus-infected cells in the context of Class I molecules of the MHC. A proposed mechanism for this interaction is suggested in Fig. 1.10. Ti molecules recognize antigen complexed with the variable regions of the Class I molecule whereas the

CD8 molecule binds to the invariant region of Class I molecules. This interaction is important both in the activation of CD8$^+$ T-lymphocytes by antigen, and in the lysis of virus-infected cells by specifically immune CTL. When CD8$^+$ cells are stimulated by specific antigen in the context of Class I molecules, these cells begin to express receptors for IL-2 which then induces proliferation and differentiation into CTL. Other lymphokines such as IL-4, IL-5 as well as IL-1 may also be important in the development of CTL.

B-lymphocytes and humoral immunity

B-lymphocytes are produced and processed in the bone marrow in mammals. Mature B-cells recirculate between the blood and lymphoid tissues although possibly not to the same extent as T-lymphocytes. Each B-lymphocyte has epitope specificity owing to the presence of specific membrane-bound receptors which in this case are antibody molecules (immunoglobulins). During an immune response, specific B-lymphocytes bind antigen molecules on the surface immunoglobulin. The antigen is then internalized, processed and presented at the cell surface in association with Class II MHC molecules. The B-lymphocyte presents antigen in this way to helper T-lymphocytes. In theory, a B-cell which recognizes one epitope on an immunogen, can present it to several T-cells with specificities for different epitopes on the same antigen.

The interaction between T- and B-cells, together with IL-1 produced by other APC leads to the proliferation and differentiation of B-lymphocytes into antibody-secreting plasma cells (Fig. 1.11). Since most immunogens, with few exceptions, contain several different antigenic determinants, several different

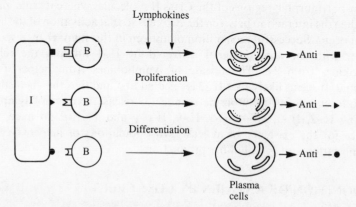

Fig. 1.11 Polyclonal B-cell response. B-lymphocytes specific for determinants on an immunogen (I) respond to the specific epitope by clonal expansion and differentiation into plasma cells secreting antibody. This process requires lymphokines supplied by activated helper T-cells.

B-lymphocytes may be stimulated, each of which will give rise to a clone of cells. The normal response is therefore said to be polyclonal.

Thus, the activation, proliferation and maturation of B-lymphocytes is therefore dependent on the presence of:

- specific antigen
- physical contact with T_H
- lymphokines secreted by T_H
- IL-1 secreted by APC

Internalization of specific antigen seems to be the trigger for the production of receptors for IL-2 and this may in turn induce the production of receptors for other important lymphokines which induce proliferation and differentiation. Amongst the lymphokines, IL-2, IL-4, IL-5 and IL-6 influence the development of antibody-secreting cells and IFN-γ can modify the class of immunoglobulin produced. Plasma cells do not normally circulate in the blood but remain in lymphoid tissues, secreting immunoglobulin which circulates via the lymphatic system into the blood.

IMMUNOGLOBULINS

In man, five different immunoglobulin (Ig) classes are found either in serum or as surface immunoglobulin on B-cells: IgM, IgG, IgA, IgE and IgD. The structure of antibody molecules is best discussed with reference to IgG (Fig. 1.12). IgG is a glycoprotein consisting of two sets of identical polypeptide chains, the heavy chains (H), with a molecular weight of 50 kDa and the light chains (L) with a

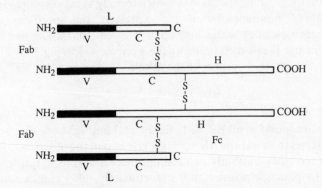

Fig. 1.12 The structure of IgG. The IgG molecule is made up of heavy (H) and light (L) chains joined by disulphide bridges. The amino-terminal ends of the chains have variable (V) amino acid sequences which together constitute the antigen-binding region (Fab). The carboxy-terminal ends are relatively constant (C), the two heavy chains making up the Fc region which determines biological activities such as placental transfer and the activation of complement.

molecular weight of 25 kDa. The chains are held together by disulphide bridges joining L to H and H to H as shown. One IgG molecule has two antigen-binding sites (Fab) at the N-terminal end of the molecules where the antibody binds a specific epitope, and an Fc region which controls biological activities of the molecule such as complement activation and placental transmission. The specificity of immunoglobulin is conferred by the unique sequence in the variable regions of the light and heavy polypeptide chains. The different classes of immunoglobulin differ in their heavy chains, where the sequence of amino acids in the constant region determines the class of the antibody. Thus, antibodies having identical V regions but different C regions will have identical specificity but will belong to a different class, and therefore may have different biological properties. The heavy chains of IgG are γ-chains, those of IgM are μ-chains, etc. Two different types of light chain occur; these are known as κ and λ and these may be combined with any of the different heavy chains so that, for example, an IgG molecule will either have $\kappa\gamma_2$ or $\lambda_2\gamma_2$ but never a mixture. In addition, some secreted immunoglobulins are polymers of the basic four chain structure. IgM, for example, exists as a polymer of five identical subunits joined together by a joining (J) chain. Table 1.4 contains a comparison of the properties of the different immunoglobulin classes.

Immature B-cells have the capacity to produce immunoglobulins of any specificity and class, having the full complement of genes for variable and constant regions. During development, however, gene rearrangements involving deletion and splicing of DNA mean that a mature B-cell is only able to produce antibody of a single specificity although, for a time, they may be capable of producing different classes of antibody. For example, the earliest B-lymphocytes express surface IgM which may later be co-expressed with IgD and/or another class. Alternatively, some B-cells may switch from IgM expression to IgA, IgG or IgE. Whatever immunoglobulins are expressed, the specificity of all immunoglobulin molecules on the same cell is identical. Surface immunoglobulin is embedded in the B-cell membrane at the Fc region, leaving Fab sites to bind antigens at the external surface of the B-cell.

The role of secreted antibody

Antibodies are found in all the body fluids. IgG and IgM are the predominant antibody classes in blood and, though IgA is found in the blood its importance is really as a secretory antibody protecting mucosal surfaces. IgE has a role in immunity to parasitic worms and, unfortunately, also causes some allergic reactions. IgD occurs frequently as a surface immunoglobulin, usually in combination with IgM but it appears only in very low concentrations in the blood. It seems likely that surface IgD is involved in antigen binding, internalization and transmission of activation signals across the B-cell membrane.

Table 1.4 Properties of human immunoglobulins

Class	Molecular weight	Serum concentration (mg/100 ml)	Complement fixation	Placental transfer	Comments
IgM	900 000	60–200	Yes	No	First antibody phylogenetically and in primary and secondary responses
IgG	150 000	800–1600	Yes (most subclasses)	Yes	Major antibody in secondary response
IgA	$(160\,000)_n$	350	No	No	Important as the antibody in secretions
IgE	180 000	0.005	No	No	Important in immune response to some parasites; responsible for some allergic reactions
IgD	180 000	3	No	No	Surface Ig on many B cells; possibly involved in antigen-induced triggering

The primary function of an antibody is to combine with an epitope and this specificity is conferred by the unique amino acid sequence in the antigen binding, or Fab regions. The molecular folding of the Fab region results in the formation of a cleft into which the epitope fits. A good 'fit', i.e. if the epitope and the binding sites have good complementary shapes, will produce a high-affinity binding (Fig. 1.13). The binding of antibody to the epitope involves a number of molecular forces including hydrophobic interactions, Van der Waals forces, and, to a lesser extent ionic interactions and hydrogen bonding. Once binding has occurred antibodies trigger destruction of the immunogen by one or more of a limited number of pathways dependent on the nature of the immunogen and the antibody class. These pathways are summarized as follows:

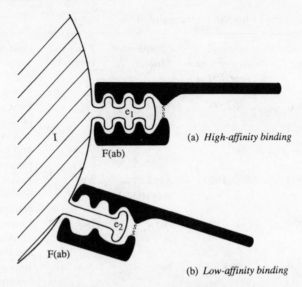

Fig. 1.13   High- and low-affinity antigen binding. The epitope fits into the 'shape' of the antigen binding site (Fab). A good fit, such as occurs between epitope e_1 of the immunogen, I, and the Fab region (only one depicted here) gives high-affinity binding. The same antibody may bind a less well 'fitting' epitope, e_2, but with much reduced affinity.

(1) The agglutination of cells, and the precipitation of soluble proteins by IgM, IgA and IgG may localize infection or render immunogens more readily phagocytosed.

(2) The binding of IgG or IgM to immunogens may activate the complement sequence which results in lysis of cellular immunogens. The complement sequence, as it is activated by antibody, is described in Fig. 1.14. The full sequence proceeds to lysis of the cell, but intermediate products of the complement sequence stimulate phagocytosis of cells and proteins.

(3) Neutrophilic PMNs have receptors for the Fc region of antigen-bound IgG which stimulates phagocytosis of immunogens.

(4) Large granular lymphocytes may kill IgG-coated cells by releasing lytic molecules on the cell. Eosinophils can kill IgG-coated parasite larvae by a related mechanism.

While the binding of antibody to an epitope is determined by the Fab region, the destruction of the immunogen, as well as a number of other biological properties, such as the serum half-life and placental transmission, are determined by sites on the Fc region, the structure of which determines the antibody class. Humoral immunity is a common feature of the immune response to bacteria and proteins. Although antibodies are produced in response to viruses and transplanted tissue, the predominant immune response towards these is T-cell-mediated.

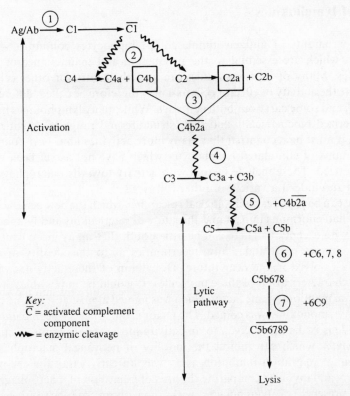

Fig. 1.14 Classical sequence for complement activation. The classical pathway of complement activation is activated by the combination of IgG or IgM with the antigen. The first component, C1, binds to the Fc regions of two adjacent IgG molecules and acquires protease activity (1), cleaving both C4 and C2 (2), each into two fragments. The larger fragments, C4b and C2a combine to form a C3 convertase (3) which cleaves C3. C3b can bind to the membrane of the target cell, and together with the C3 convertase, cleaves C5. Each enzymic step represents considerable amplification of the response. C5b also binds to the cell membrane and the subsequent components, C6, 7, 8 and 6 molecules of C9 add on to form the 'membrane attack complex' (MAC). This hydrophobic complex pushes out a hole in the cell membrane. The activation of a single C1 molecule may result in thousands of MAC over the cell membrane, leading to lysis.

The alternative pathway, not depicted here, is activated by bacterial lipopolysaccharide from bacterial cell walls, without the involvement of antibody. This pathway, which is actually an amplification loop, results also in the production of a C3 convertase and its products feed into the lytic pathway.

Phagocytes have receptors for C3b, and the subsequent binding facilitates uptake of the immunogen. Other complement components, such as C2a, C3a and C5a, may stimulate inflammation and/or are chemotactic for polymorphonuclear leukocytes.

Role of lymphokines

The supernatants of antigen-stimulated T-lymphocytes contain a variety of proteins which are essential to the production and maintenance of immune responses. Many of these molecules are growth factors for other cells, some stimulate the activity of effector cells and may therefore be called 'differentiation factors', and some carry out both activities. While many lymphokines have been characterized biochemically and their structure and range of activities is well known, it must be recognized that many more activities have been found in the supernatants of stimulated lymphocytes which have not as yet been very well characterized. These include factors with activity towards macrophages, polymorphs and indeed a variety of other cell types.

There can be few areas of biological research in which the new gene technology has not had enormous impact and the study of interleukins and lymphokines is certainly no exception. There can be little doubt that many more lymphokines will be characterized and many uncertainties as to the identity of different activities resolved in the near future. Discussion of these activities will await further characterization of these molecules. It would be impossible, though, to omit from mentioning one factor which was named almost at the same time that the term 'lymphokine' was coined. The factor is the *macrophage inhibitory factor* (MIF). This is the name given to an activity in the supernatants of stimulated lymphocytes which can inhibit the motility of peritoneal macrophages. The macrophage migration inhibition assay was an early assay for cell-mediated immunity and involved comparing the area of migration of macrophages grown in the presence of lymphocytes with or without specific antigen. If the lymphocytes were sensitized, contact with antigen resulted in the release of MIF which inhibited migration. It seems ironic that one of the earliest activities named has not yet been fully characterized. In fact several proteins, including IFNγ, appear to have some MIF activity.

The lymphokines and interleukins which will be discussed in this book are those which have been characterized and the genes cloned and sequenced. A brief summary of the role of these lymphokines and interleukins is given in Table 1.5, but more comprehensive discussions will be found in future chapters.

MECHANISM OF ACTION OF LYMPHOKINES

Lymphokines act on target cells by binding to a specific cell receptor. Following binding, biochemical changes take place which result in a signal being transmitted across the membrane of the cell and into the cytoplasm. Since the lymphokine has different effects on different target cells, it is possible that the signal transmission mechanism changes, or that the cell is in some way pre-programmed to behave in a particular way on receipt of the signal. The nature of lymphokine receptors – few have been biochemically characterized – and their mechanism of action is poorly understood. Although little is known about the

Table 1.5 Function of well-characterized interleukins

Protein	Function(s)
IL-1	Stimulates T-cells; stimulates inflammation, fever; tumoricidal
IL-2	Supports proliferation and differentiation of T- and B-lymphocytes; increases the activity of NK cell
IL-3	Stimulates growth and differentiation of bone marrow stem cells (gives rise to blood cells); a growth factor for mast cells
IL-4	Mast cell growth factor; T-cell growth factor; growth and differentiation factor for B cells; stimulates IgE production
IL-5	Eosinophil growth and fifferentiation factor; B-cell growth and differentiation factor (stimulates IgA)
IL-6	Stimulatory factor for B cells; produces inflammation
IL-7	Production of B-cell precursors in bone marrow
IFN-γ	Antiviral; activates macrophages; stimulates NK cells; may inhibit antibody production or alter the class of antibody produced
TNF	Inflammatory, antitumour effects, causes 'toxic shock'

biochemical events involved in signal transduction and transmission across the membrane, it is generally assumed that the effects of lymphokines are mediated through one of a relatively few biochemical pathways which are known to mediate the effects of hormones on cells. These pathways involve the use of intrinsic membrane proteins which transmit the message across the membrane, and small molecules, known as 'second messengers' which are able to diffuse in the cytoplasm and thus transmit the signal inside the cell. What follows is simply a discussion of some of these pathways which *may* be involved in lymphokine interaction at the cell surface. What little is known about individual lymphokines will be discussed in the ensuing chapters.

Signal transduction and the second messenger hypothesis

The ability of a particular cell to respond to a messenger molecule such as a hormone (or, in this case, a lymphokine) depends on whether or not that cell expresses the correct receptor. It is in the possession of the correct receptors that the specificity of the response resides. Within the cell membrane are a series of integral membrane proteins, the function of which is to transmit the signal across the membrane. These proteins can undergo reversible changes in conformation and by doing so can act as a signal transducing mechanism. Interaction of the ligand with the receptor causes a conformational change in one protein which then causes a similar change in another protein and so on (Fig. 1.15). At the end of this sequence of conformational changes the signal is transmitted to the second messengers, small molecules or ions which diffuse within the cytoplasm and propagate the signal throughout the cell. The proteins which form the

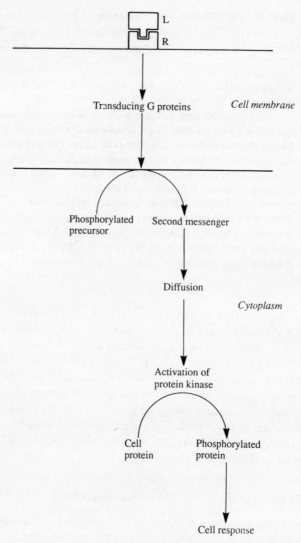

Fig. 1.15 Signal transduction across the cell membrane. Lymphokines, like hormones, interact with specific receptors in the cell membrane of target cells. The binding may trigger off a series of events, resulting in transmission of the signal across the membrane. Binding of the ligand (L) to the receptor (R), causes conformational changes in G proteins which pass the signal through the membrane. At the cytoplasmic surface, the G proteins activate an 'amplifier' protein which converts a phosphorylated precursor molecule into a 'second messenger' which diffuses through the cytoplasm. The second messenger activates a protein kinase which phosphorylates a cell protein, resulting in the cellular response.

transduction pathway are G (guanine nucleotide regulatory) proteins, which bind GTP before activation. The G proteins activate an enzyme on the inner face of the cell membrane which converts precursor molecules into the active second messenger. The second messenger may act directly by binding to cell proteins and causing activation or, more commonly, by activating another enzyme, a protein kinase, which phosphorylates proteins, induces changes in conformation and hence in activity.

At least two major pathways have been discovered. In the first pathway, the second messenger is cyclic AMP (cAMP). The second pathway, the PIP pathway, uses a combination of calcium ions, inositol triphosphate and diacylglycerol, the latter being derived from membrane phospholipids.

Cyclic AMP pathways. This pathway can result in stimulation or inhibition of an activity depending on which type of receptors (stimulatory or inhibitory) are engaged and, hence, which G proteins are activated. Two G proteins are involved: a stimulatory (G_s) and an inhibitory (G_i). The transduction pathway results in activation of adenylate cyclase which converts ATP into cAMP. Cyclic AMP in turn activates protein kinase-A.

PIP pathway. This pathway can only act in a stimulatory capacity. Signal transduction via G proteins results in the activation of a phosphodiesterase which converts phosphatidylinositol-4,5-biphosphate into diacylglycerol (DAG) and inositol triphosphate (IP3). IP3 is involved in mobilization of calcium ions from storage in the endoplasmic reticulum and these ions can activate a protein kinase following binding to the protein calmodulin. Diacylglycerol remaining in the membrane can activate another protein kinase (protein kinase-C) which can also activate cell proteins by the process of phosphorylation.

Summary

The specificity of the immune response resides in small lymphocytes which have receptors for, and respond to, a specific antigenic determinant. Two different populations of small lymphocytes, namely B-cells and T-cells are responsible for humoral and cell-mediated immunity, respectively. The function and phenotype of these lymphocytes is dependent on their developmental 'processing'. Other T-lymphocytes have regulatory functions and the helper T-cell in particular produces lymphokines which are essential for the antigen-induced proliferation and differentiation of B-cells and cytotoxic/suppressor T-cells. The production of lymphokines by helper T-cells is antigen-induced and is dependent on the presence of antigen-presenting cells as well as IL-1 which they release. The major histocompatibility complex exerts control over these reactions by specifying the synthesis of cell-surface glycoproteins which must be recognized by the T-lymphocytes. Non-specific effector cells such as macrophages and NK cells may be recruited into a specific immune response by lymphokines released after antigenic stimulation.

References

Berridge, M. J. (1985). 'The molecular basis of communication within the cell', *Scientific American* **253**, p. 124.

Dale, M. M. and Foreman, J. C. (1989). *Textbook of Immunopharmacology*, 2nd edn. Oxford, Blackwell Scientific Publications.

Playfair, J. H. L. (1987). *Immunology at a Glance*, 4th edn. Oxford. Blackwell Scientific Publications.

Roitt, I. (1988). *Essential Immunology*, 6th edn. Oxford, Blackwell Scientific Publications.

Roitt, I. M., Brostoff, J. and Male, D. K. (1989). *Immunology*, 2nd edn. London. Gower Medical Publishing.

Zouhair Atassi, M. (1984). *Molecular Immunology*. New York, Marcel Dekker.

2

Production of Lymphokines

Introduction

The term 'lymphokine' was coined by Dumonde, in the 1960s, and for several years much research time and effort was expended in determining the range of activities which could be promoted by supernatants of activated lymphocytes. The presence of factors such as MIF in the supernatants of lymphocytes cultured with antigen was used as a test for cell-mediated immunity, just as the presence of specific antibody indicated humoral immunity. The discovery of T-cell growth factor (IL-2) in 1976, marked a turning point in the study of lymphokines which were shown to have fundamentally important roles in the development of an immune response, in addition to their role as the effector products of cell-mediated immunity. For several years also, progress in the biochemical characterization of these molecules was hampered both by the inability to obtain sufficient quantities of pure proteins from stimulated lymphocytes, and by the painstaking and laborious techniques which were then available for sequencing proteins. Until the last decade, our knowledge of the structural properties of these molecules and their receptors consisted of little more than the molecular weights and susceptibility to heat, pH and proteolytic enzymes.

During the last 10 years, the study of lymphokines has brought tremendous advances and major scientific discoveries are being made at rapidly decreasing intervals of time. There are several reasons, of course, for this upsurge of activity. First and foremost must be the remarkable progress in the techniques of molecular biology which have come about in that time and which have allowed both the biochemical characterization of proteins which would otherwise have taken many years and the production of pure lymphokines on a hitherto unimaginable scale. It has been estimated, for example, that more human IL-2 has now been produced by recombinant DNA technology than has ever been produced as a result of immune responses occurring *in vivo* in the history of mankind! In addition, the clinical potential for some of these molecules has generated much interest in research. For example, IL-2 and IFN-γ have both been tested as potential antitumour agents, while IL-3 may be useful for stimulating haemopoiesis in patients whose bone marrow is depleted, for example, by cytotoxic drugs used for cancer chemotherapy.

In technological terms, though, molecular biology has not been solely responsible for the 'lymphokine revolution' and it is the intention of this chapter to discuss other techniques which are available both for producing lymphokines and (in Chapter 3) for analysing their activities. This will enable the present work to be set in an historical context and will allow a discussion of the particular uses of these other techniques. The ability to clone lymphocytes in culture, for example, has enabled the cellular origins of lymphokines to be ascertained whereas the production of T-cell hybridomas can also help to elucidate the chromosomal location of lymphokine genes.

Production of lymphokines

Cells which can be used to produce lymphokines (Table 2.1) *in vitro* fall into one of the following categories:

(a)　Stimulated T-lymphocytes
(b)　T-cell hybridomas
(c)　Constitutive or inducible cell lines
(d)　Prokaryotic or eukaryotic cells containing lymphokine-specific recombinant DNA

Of these four, only the last can realistically produce sufficient quantities of these proteins to satisfy the present and future commercial and clinical requirements. However, the ability to produce these proteins by recombinant DNA technology is, in the first instance, dependent on research in the other three: For example, in order to produce a lymphokine-specific DNA for insertion into bacteria, it is necessary to isolate specific mRNA and to do this one must first ascertain which cells produce it, how they can be maximally stimulated and the kinetics of the response. With the exception of IL-1 and TNF-α, all the proteins discussed in

Table 2.1　List of some useful cells lines producing particular lymphokines

Lymphokine	Culture	Derivation
IL-2	MLA-144	Gibbon lymphoblastoid line
IL-3	WEHI-3B	Mouse myelomonocytic leukaemia
TNF-α	HL60	Human myelomonocytic line
TNF-β	RPMI 1788	Human B-lymphoblastoid line

later chapters of this book can be produced by T-lymphocytes (which is not to say that other cells are not capable of producing them). The first two categories, then, do not apply to IL-1 and TNF-α which are the products of antigen-presenting cells. The production of IL-1 can, however, be induced in APC by particular treatments and these are discussed in Chapter 4.

TISSUE CULTURE

With the exception of recombinant DNA technology utilizing prokaryotic cells or yeasts, the production of lymphokines necessitates the culture of mammalian cells. Tissue culture of such cells is brought about by growing them in defined media supplemented with serum, usually newborn calf or fetal bovine, which contains essential factors for growth. The use of cultured mammalian cells for the production of lymphokines has a number of drawbacks not the least of which is the possibility of infection. Gross infection with bacteria or yeasts is easily spotted since the contaminating cells quickly outgrow the mammalian cells which have a considerably longer doubling time. What is more of a problem is sub-lethal contamination, principally with *Mycoplasma* and viruses which may slow down the growth rate of cells without necessarily killing them and which, moreover, may prove to be a problem if the cell products are to be used for injection. All tissue cultures used to produce lymphokines should be routinely tested for *Mycoplasma* infection which can sometimes be resolved by use of appropriate antibiotics. Sera which are obtained from commercial sources are tested both for *Mycoplasma* infection and for their ability to support the growth of cells because considerable batch variation can occur and some samples can, for unknown reasons, be poor at supporting growth of cells. Because of the variability between batches of serum and the high cost of animal sera many laboratories are developing and using serum-free media. These are formulations of media in which the serum content is replaced by a selection of essential factors and hormones such as transferrin, insulin and bovine serum albumin. On the whole, serum-free media formulations appear to be successful and, in addition to the more predictable aspects of their use, they are also free of bacterial endotoxin and require the use of fewer living animals.

STIMULATION OF LYMPHOCYTES

Source of lymphocytes

In order to stimulate lymphocytes into releasing lymphokines it is first necessary to obtain reasonably pure populations of T-lymphocytes so as to reduce contamination with the products of other cell types. On the other hand, lymphocyte populations which have been totally depleted of monocytes will not produce lymphokines either so that a balance is necessary to maximize production. Human lymphocytes may be conveniently isolated from peripheral

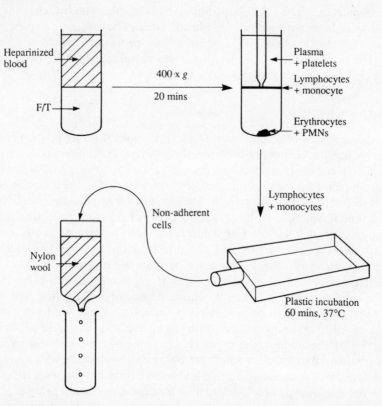

Fig. 2.1 Preparation of lymphocytes from blood. Blood is heparinized to prevent clotting and carefully layered onto a Ficoll/Triosil (F/T) mixture with a precise density of 1.077 g/ml. When the tubes are centrifuged, the cells with a higher density than this (erythrocytes and PMNs) pellet at the bottom of the tube. Lymphocytes and monocytes, which both have a density <1.077 g/ml, are found at the interface between the plasma and the Ficoll/Triosil mixture. Further purification can be achieved by incubating the mixture in plastic tissue culture flasks for 60 min. The monocytes adhere strongly to the plastic. The B-lymphocytes can be removed by incubation on nylon wool columns, which also removes any remaining monocytes. The T-cells emerging from the column have purities of 95–99%.

blood by density-gradient centrifugation (Fig. 2.1). The volume of blood which can be obtained from small animals such as rodents and mice precludes the use of peripheral blood, and here solid lymphoid tissues, especially the spleen, are the best alternative source. The spleen is easily dispersed into single cells by gentle homogenization and the suspension can be fractionated on Ficoll-Triosil gradients as for whole blood.

The cells obtained from these gradients are a mixture of T- and B-lymphocytes and monocytes. T-lymphocytes can be further purified by incubation in plastic

(a) *Immunofluorescence*

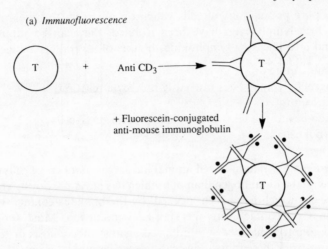

(b) *Fluorescence-activated cell sorter* (FACS)

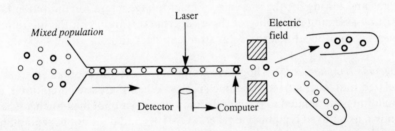

Fig. 2.2 Separation of T- and B-cells by immunofluorescence. (a) A monoclonal antibody to the CD3 surface protein will bind to T-cells only. Since the monoclonal antibody is a mouse immunoglobulin, incubation with a fluorescein-conjugated anti-mouse immunoglobulin antibody, will ensure that T-cells fluoresce in UV light. (b) Fluorescent-labelled T-lymphocytes can be separated from non-labelled B-cells in a fluorescence-activated cell sorter. Since cells are illuminated with a laser beam and the degree of fluorescence measured by a detector, connected to a computer. The fluorescing and non-fluorescing cells are assigned a positive or negative electric charge and passed through an electric field where, depending on the charge, they are deflected into two collecting tubes.

tissue culture flasks to which monocytes adhere, while B-lymphocytes are removed by isolation on nylon wool columns. Alternatively, T-cells can be selectively stained by immunofluorescence using a monoclonal antibody to a T-cell-specific marker such as OKT3 (see Chapter 1) followed by separation on a fluorescence-activated cell sorter (FACS) (Fig. 2.2). Although these machines are not a routine feature of immunology laboratories, the capital expense and running costs being, for many, prohibitively expensive, their use can provide extremely pure populations of cells which do not seem to be harmed by the process. Once lymphocytes have been isolated, they can be stimulated into mitosis and into releasing lymphokines by one of several agents including:

(1)   Specific antigen
(2)   Allogeneic lymphocytes (mixed lymphocyte reaction)
(3)   Plant lectins
(4)   Antibodies to the CD3 cell surface protein on T-cells
(5)   Phorbol esters

Specific antigen.   An immunized animal has larger numbers of cells capable of responding to the immunogen than one which has never previously encountered it. These cells, which have been 'primed' by the previous contact, will release lymphokines on contact with the specific immunogen. Most people in the developed countries have been immunized against tuberculosis or tetanus and lymphocytes from these individuals can release lymphokines *in vitro* following incubation with tuberculin or tetanus toxoid. Indeed, one of the first *in vitro* tests for cell mediated immunity (CMI) involved taking the supernatants from such systems and testing for the presence of macrophage migration inhibition factor (MIF) by assessing the ability of these supernatants to inhibit the migration of guinea-pig peritoneal macrophages from capillary tubes.

Allogeneic lymphocytes.   Allogeneic lymphocytes are those obtained from two unrelated individuals from the same species. When these are co-cultured, each population is stimulated to proliferate and release lymphokines. Such a reaction is known as a mixed lymphocyte reaction (MLR) and does not depend on prior immunization (more properly the MLR is a mixed *leukocyte* reaction since the presence of monocytes is essential). If one population is prevented from dividing by prior treatment with mitomycin-C or by irradiation, a one-way reaction will occur, the treated cells acting as a stimulator for the second (responder) population. During an MLR, lymphokines such as IL-2 and IFN-γ are released from the responder population. Again, such supernatants can only be used for crude lymphokine preparations, and are not convenient for investigations which require larger amounts of pure mediators.

Plant lectins.   When lymphocytes are stimulated with specific immunogen only those cells with specific receptors for the immunogen will respond, the degree of response being dependent on the extent of immunity in the individual. Plant lectins such as phytohaemagglutinin (PHA) and concanavalin-A (Con-A) are proteins which bind to glycosyl residues present on the surface of lymphocytes and mimic the effect of antigen in stimulating proliferation. The effects of lectins are often confined to one population of lymphocytes so that pokeweed mitogen (PWM) stimulates B-lymphocytes while PHA and Con-A stimulate T-cells. The supernatants of PHA and Con-A stimulated lymphocytes have been used extensively as crude source of lymphokines. IL-2, for example, was first discovered as a factor in the supernatants of PHA-treated lymphocytes, which could support the growth of activated T-cells in culture. Such supernatants can provide a cocktail of lymphokines which can also be used to support antibody production by antigen-stimulated B-lymphocytes *in vitro*. However, these crude preparations have seldom been used as a source of lymphokines for biochemical characterization or for clinical use, since an individual lymphokine is present in such small amounts and would require extensive biochemical purification before a single activity could be attributed unequivocally to it.

Antibodies to the CD3 molecule. The CD3 molecule is present on the surface of all mature T-lymphocytes where it is associated with the epitope-specific T-cell receptor to form the T-cell receptor complex. The role of CD3 is to transmit an activation signal across the T-cell membrane when specific antigen has bound to the T-cell receptor. Monoclonal antibodies to CD3 can mimic the effect of specific antigen, possibly by cross-linking CD3 molecules and causing membrane perturbations. Thus, anti-CD3 results in T-cell proliferation and triggers the release of lymphokines. Such activation has recently been used for studying cells which produce lymphokines. For example, CD3 activated cells have been stained by immunofluorescence, using monoclonal antibodies to individual differentiation antigens and antibodies to IFN-γ. Thus, a cell which was shown to be synthesizing IFN-γ could be identified by a phenotypic marker. In this way, it was shown that both CD4$^+$ and CD8$^+$ cells, as well as the non-T natural killer (NK) cells were capable of producing this interferon.

Phorbol esters (PMA). Phorbol esters such as phorbol myristate acetate (PMA) and 12-O-tetradecanoylphorbol-13-acetate (TPA) are potent stimulators of lymphocyte mitosis and lymphokine release. These esters will also enhance the release of lymphokines from T-cell hybridomas. Phorbol esters are useful agents for helping to analyse the immune response *in vitro* but they are also tumour-promoting agents so that it is unlikely that lymphokines induced in this way would ever be used for the treatment of human disease.

In conclusion, then, the production of lymphokines can be induced in 'bulk' cultures of lymphocytes *in vitro* and different activities can be identified and to some extent purified. One of the major problems associated with the production of lymphokines by all of these methods is that any desired factor is swamped by the multitude of other factors which are co-stimulated. Thus, extensive purification may be necessary to provide a 'pure' sample. Moreover, most lymphokines are active at protein concentrations of $\leqslant 1$ ng/ml so that even minimal contamination of one lymphokine with another may have misleading results, especially since recent work has shown that lymphokines often have overlapping activities and act synergistically. In addition, the presence of the original stimulatory substance such as PHA or PMA may be highly undesirable.

Some of the preparations outlined above have provided limited information concerning the types of cells which produce individual lymphokines, and have also furnished crude lymphokine preparations which can be useful in the laboratory. For example, lyophilized supernatants from lectin-stimulated lymphocytes are currently marketed for use in monoclonal antibody production. The usual method for the production of monoclonal antibodies involves extensive immunization of mice which may take several months in total. A quicker method involves stimulating mouse spleen cells with antigen *in vitro* in the presence of a cocktail of lymphokines. This technique is particularly useful in the production of human monoclonal antibodies where immunization of individuals, possibly with potentially harmful antigens, can be avoided and where isolation of antibody-producing cells from the blood of immunized individuals is difficult. Whatever method is used for the production of monoclonal antibodies, the initial growth of B-cell hybridomas has been shown to be dependent on a lymphokine initially called hybridoma and plasmacytoma growth factor (HPGF), and now known as interleukin 6 (IL-6).

CLONING OF LYMPHOCYTES

One of the most remarkable features of the specific immune response is that an individual lymphocyte will respond only to a single epitope and, on appropriate stimulation with that epitope, will respond by clonal expansion (see Chapter 1). Immune responses are polyclonal in nature in that most immunogens contain different epitopes which stimulate lymphocytes bearing different receptors. The responding lymphocytes may be B-cells, in which case the products of clonal expansion are antibody-secreting plasma cells; T-helper cells which proliferate and release lymphokines capable of 'helping' B-cells or of inducing delayed hypersensitivity, or it may be a potentially cytotoxic T-lymphocyte.

Since the early 1980s it has become possible not only to grow antigen- or mitogen-stimulated lymphocytes in 'bulk', i.e. polyclonal, culture, but also to isolate and grow up stimulated lymphocytes so that they form a clone of cells in isolation from other antigen-specific lymphocytes. Such cloning methods have been used to examine the cells involved in the immune response and the factors that they produce. Certain clones and/or their products may be investigated for their interaction with other cell clones/products and synergistic effects noted. The cloning of lymphocytes is discussed here principally in relation to T-cells although in many cases they could equally apply to B-lymphocytes or other cells generally. Lymphocytes may be cloned either by the method of limiting dilution, or by the use of soft agar cultures.

Limiting dilution analysis

In this technique (Fig. 2.3) lymphocytes are stimulated by culture with mitogens or with specific antigens and are 'seeded' into multi-well tissue culture plates at very low cell densities, from 10 cells per well down to 0.3 cell per well (i.e. 3 cells

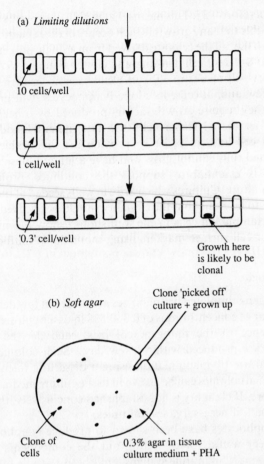

(a) *Limiting dilutions*

10 cells/well

1 cell/well

'0.3' cell/well

Growth here
is likely to be
clonal

Clone 'picked off'
culture + grown up

(b) *Soft agar*

Clone of
cells

0.3% agar in tissue
culture medium + PHA

Fig. 2.3 Cloning of cells. (a) Limiting dilutions. Activated T-cell suspensions are diluted to very low cell densities and plated into the wells of plastic microtitre trays. ('0.3' cell/well represents 3 cells every 10 wells.) At very low cell densities, the growth of cells in a well where 37% of wells have no growth is, according to the Poisson distribution, very likely to be clonal. Such low cell densities require 'feeder cells' which have been irradiated to prevent growth. (b) Soft agar cloning. Single T-lymphocytes, activated with PHA, will produce colonies in semi-solid agar. These colonies can be 'picked up' from the agar using a dissection microscope and re-cloned to ensure clonality.

every 10 wells). The number of clones which grow in each well can be related to the number of wells in which no growth occurs by the following formula which is derived from Poisson distribution analysis:

$$F_0 = e^{-u}$$

where F_0 is the fraction of wells with no growth, e is the exponential (2.718282) and u is the number of clonal precursor cells per well. For monoclonal growth,

$u = 1$ and F_0 is therefore 0.37. This means that if 37% of the wells show no growth, it is highly probable that any growth which occurs in the remaining wells is due to clonal outgrowth (i.e. all the cells are derived from a single progenitor). Thus cells are plated out at different cell densities and clones assumed to occur at that cell plating density which results in 37% of wells have no growth.

In practice, few animal cells, let alone lymphocytes, will grow at such low densities since they require growth factors produced by other cells. It is usual therefore to add irradiated 'feeder' cells such as peripheral blood lymphocytes or lymphoblastoid cell lines in order to provide the favourable conditions for growth. Irradiated cells cannot grow and have a limited lifespan in culture. In addition, IL-2 is essential to support the continued proliferation of T-lymphocytes in culture. Cultures which arise in wells seeded at the correct density are highly likely to be clones but the clonality should be checked by a number of methods. For example, all cells in the well should show a similar 'phenotype' when stained for cell surface markers using monoclonal antibodies.

Cloning in soft agar

Mitogen or antigen-stimulated lymphocytes are seeded at low densities into 'soft' or semi-solid agar at concentrations of 0.3–0.5% in tissue culture medium. In the continued presence of the mitogen, colonies, each derived from a single progenitor cell, are produced within a few days. Such colonies can be easily 'picked off' a culture by manipulation using a dissecting microscope and fine pipettes. Individual colonies can be grown in tissue culture medium and tested for clonality as before. If clonality is not established conclusively, then the cells can easily be re-cloned, if necessary, several times.

Cloned T-lymphocytes have been shown to produce lymphokines and have proved to be very useful for dissecting out the components of an immune response. For example, in murine systems it has been possible to distinguish two types of helper T-lymphocyte (T_{H1} and T_{H2}) which, although identical in terms of cell-surface markers, actually produce mutually exclusive lymphokines. T_{H1} for example produces IL-2 and IFN-γ whereas T_{H2} produces IL-4 and IL-5. The clones, and supernatants obtained from them, have been used to analyse the cellular interactions which may take place, in a relatively simple *in vitro* system and are also useful for establishing synergistic and antagonistic effects of different supernatants. They are not, however, particularly useful for the large-scale production of lymphokines, which is generally achieved by recombinant DNA technology.

T-CELL HYBRIDOMAS

Attempts to produce hybridomas from stimulated T-cells fused to cancer cells followed the highly successful production, by Kohler and Milstein in 1975, of a B-cell hybridoma making monoclonal antibody to sheep erythrocytes. B-cell hybridomas, produced by the fusion of antibody-producing mouse spleen cells

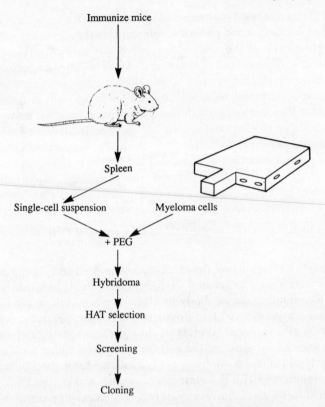

Immunize mice

Spleen

Single-cell suspension   Myeloma cells

+ PEG

Hybridoma

HAT selection

Screening

Cloning

Fig. 2.4 Production of B-cell hybridomas. Mice immunized with the appropriate antigen make specific antibody. The spleen is a convenient source of the cells which make the antibody. After several immunizations, to boost the response, the mice are sacrificed and the spleens removed and mildly homogenized to dissociate the cells. The single cells are fused with a mouse myeloma adapted to tissue culture and selected in HAT medium. Hybridomas are screened for the appropriate antibody and positive cultures are cloned.

with cells from a culture-adapted mouse myeloma, resulted in a hybridoma which could be cloned, which had the growth characteristics of the myeloma cells, and which produced homogeneous antibody of the requisite specificity. Since 1975, monoclonal antibody technology has become well established and it is now possible to produce these antibodies to any immunogens and haptens which can be linked to a carrier protein such as BSA prior to immunization.

A brief outline of the method of monoclonal antibody production will be given in order to understand problems associated with the production of T-cell hybridomas. The majority of monoclonal antibodies are produced in mice. Briefly, mice are hyperimmunized with the immunogen in order to establish a good antibody response (Fig. 2.4). The immunization protocol may involve several injections, often over a period of weeks or months. When a good antibody

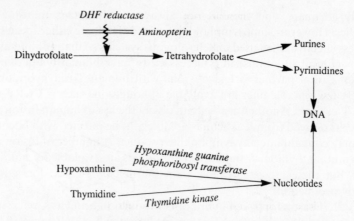

Fig. 2.5   HAT selection. (Aminopterin blocks the action of DHF reductase.)

response has been established, the animals are sacrificed and the spleen removed. It is a relatively simple procedure to disaggregate the spleen into a single-cell suspension containing the antibody-producing cells and these are fused with a mutant mouse myeloma cell line (frequently the NS1 line) using polyethylene-glycol (PEG) as a fusogen. Hybrids of the spleen cells and myeloma cells are positively selected by growing the cultures in hypoxanthine aminopterin and thymidine (HAT) medium. Aminopterin is a folic acid antagonist which prevents growth by interfering with the synthesis of purines and pyrimidines, and hence DNA. Most cells have salvage pathway enzymes: hypoxanthine guanine phosphoribosyl transferase (HGPRT) and thymidine kinase (TK) whereby the cells bypass the effect of aminopterin if they are supplied with the substrates hypoxanthine and thymidine. The mutant myeloma is selected so that it is deficient in either HGPRT or TK (NS1 is HGPRT⁻) and thus it is unable to grow in HAT medium. Hybrids produced from myeloma and spleen cells are able to grow by virtue of the enzyme supplied by the spleen cells which have the normal complement of salvage pathway enzymes (Fig. 2.5). After a few weeks in culture, all myeloma cells have died and the hybrids can be cloned in normal tissue culture medium. In the initial stages of growth, the hybridomas are genetically unstable and may shed chromosomes in a manner which is semi-random. However, after several weeks in culture a stable phenotype is achieved and at this stage hybridomas secreting the correct antibody can be classed as stable in terms of chromosome content over an indefinite period of time (some hybridomas produced in the late 1970s are still stable some 10 years later).

It is possible to produce T-cell hybridomas which secrete lymphokines *in vitro* but several problems not encountered with B-cell hybridomas are inherent in the use of T-lymphocytes. For example, since murine systems have been the best established, the majority of monoclonal antibodies are mouse immunoglobulins. For many purposes, even for some clinical situations, mouse antibodies are perfectly adequate, and there is not always an advantage to using human antibodies. However, some lymphokines, such as IL-4, are either species-specific or are less effective when used in heterologous systems so that, for human studies (and for clinical situations), it is necessary to have human lymphokines. The choice of fusion partner is less obvious with human T-cell hybridomas and relatively few suitable lines are available although one such is CCRF-CEM, a human T-cell line. Another problem involving the use of human fusion partners is that cells derived from leukaemias are likely to be infected with latent viruses which may contaminate any lymphokine product. A number of fusion partners such as mutant thymomas and T-cell lymphomas are available for murine T-cell hybrids but these are less reliable than the myelomas used for monoclonal antibody production.

One other reason for T-cell hybridoma production being less well established than monoclonal antibody production has been the fact that, since 1976, it has been possible to clone T-cells without hybridization in the presence of IL-2 and specific antigen or mitogen. Although T-cell hybridomas have the advantage that they do not require exogenous growth factors, they are often less stable in terms of phenotype than cultured T-cells or B-cell hybridomas.

Once a fusion partner has been established the production of T-cell hybridomas is similar to that for monoclonal antibodies. Lymphocytes can be obtained from animals which have been immunized with reagents known to induce cell mediated immunity or delayed hypersensitivity, for example by skin painting with a skin-sensitizing chemical such as picryl chloride or fluoro-dinitrobenzene. T-cells isolated from the spleen, lymph node or blood can be fused to a suitable thymoma and the hybrid selected by a suitable technique. The HAT selection may not be suitable for T-cell hybridomas because thymidine can inhibit the growth of T-cells. Once hybridomas have been selected and cloned, administration of specific antigen or mitogen is required to stimulate lymphokine secretion. Unlike B-cell hybridomas, frequent re-cloning of T-cell hybridomas may be necessary to maintain lymphokine-secreting capacity. Human T-cell hybridomas have been produced which have been shown to secrete immunoregulatory molecules such as IL-2 and various B-cell growth and differentiation factors.

CONSTITUTIVE CELL LINES

The availability of cell lines producing particular lymphokines will be covered in individual chapters. Such cell lines have been of great value in obtaining a supply of lymphokines without, usually, the degree of contamination with other molecules which is usual in cultures of stimulated lymphocytes. Moreover, the amount of an individual lymphokine which is produced may be considerably higher in such a cell line. However, care must be taken in interpreting results obtained from using a crude extract of a conditioned medium. For example, the gibbon MLA 144 cell line has been used extensively as a source of IL-2; only recently has it been established that this cell line also produces IL-3 constitutively. Other cell lines are available which produce a lymphokine only after stimulation with phorbol esters. Examples include the JURKAT line, derived from a T-cell leukaemia, which produces IL-2 and the EL4 mouse thymoma line which produces IL-5 and IL-2 after treatment with phorbol myristate acetate.

RECOMBINANT DNA TECHNOLOGY

The production of lymphokines and interleukins by recombinant DNA technology is nowadays the only realistic way in which large amounts of the pure proteins can be produced for pharmaceutical purposes. These methods have largely superseded those which rely on the stimulation of lymphocytes in tissue culture. Recombinant DNA technology involves the isolation and/or the production of DNA which codes for a particular eukaryotic protein and the insertion of this DNA into another cell type where it can be expressed.

Recipient cells

The recipient cell type should ideally have a fast growth rate under the normal conditions obtaining in tissue cultures with no specialist requirements for unusual growth factors, etc. Both prokaryotes and eukaryotes are suitable recipients and human lymphokine genes have been inserted in *E. coli*, yeast cells and mammalian eukaryotic cells such as Chinese Hamster Ovary (CHO) cells. Bacteria have a much shorter generation time than mammalian cells and require relatively simple media for growth *in vitro*. However, lymphokines produced in prokaryotes do not have the range of post-translational modifications which is a frequent feature of eukaryotic proteins.

When proteins are produced in eukaryotes a variety of such modifications may affect the activity of the final product and these include the addition of carbohydrate (glycosylation), lipid (myristylation), phosphorylation and sulphation. In addition, folding of the molecule may influence the physico-chemical properties of the product. An example of this might be the glycosylated form of IFN-γ which has either one or two glycosylation sites filled with an oligosaccharide side-chain. These side-chains culminate in sialic acid residues which, if removed, result in the interferon being preferentially taken up into the liver of injected animals. Bacterial products may also be contaminated with endotoxin which is a powerful inducer of fever (pyrogen).

Yeasts are eukaryotic cells, with the potential for post-translational modification, and with the growth rates of bacteria. However, it is often found that the recipient cell, though capable of glycosylation, modifies the proteins in a manner which differs from the original cell.

Production of recombinant lymphokine

The sequence of events in the production of recombinant lymphokine is outlined as follows and in Fig. 2.6.

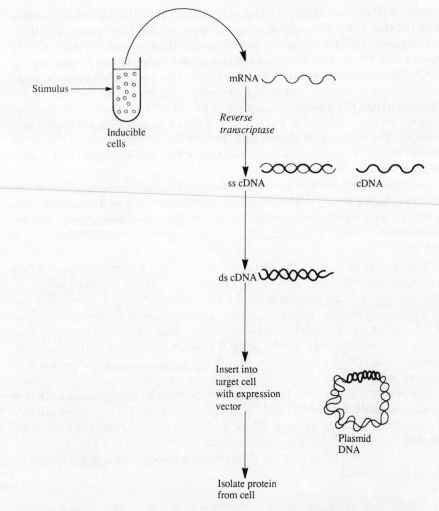

Fig. 2.6 Production of a recombinant lymphokine. Messenger RNA is extracted from cells known to produce a particular lymphokine after stimulation. A cDNA copy is made using the retroviral enzyme reverse transcriptase and the DNA inserted into target cells with an expressed vector. The cells are cultured and the protein extracted. (ss cDNA = single stranded cDNA, ds cDNA = double stranded cDNA.)

1. Isolation of mRNA. Cells are obtained which are known to produce the required lymphokine upon appropriate stimulation. Once a cell line has been chosen, the kinetics of the response must be determined in order to establish the time of optimum specific mRNA synthesis. The proportion of newly synthesized mRNA which is specific for the required lymphokine is therefore determined by the cell itself and the stimulus. For example, T-cells stimulated with PHA will contain mRNA for a range of lymphokines whereas JURKAT cells stimulated with phorbol esters will contain a high proportion of mRNA coding for IL-2.

Eukaryotic mRNA has a polyadenylated (PolyA) tail consisting of 50–200 bases at the 3′ end of the molecule and this property can be used to separate the mRNA from the bulk of the RNA in the cells. The 'bulk' RNA preparation is passed down a column containing thymidine oligomers linked to cellulose. Polyadenylated RNA binds to oligothymidine and, at high salt concentrations, is retained on the column. The mRNA can be eluted using a buffer of lower ionic strength. The recovery of all polyadenylated RNA by this technique can be as high as 90% although the proportion of total RNA which is adenylated is only around 5%.

In order to identify specific mRNA fractions further (and therefore to cut down on future work), mRNA fractions can be injected into *Xenopus* oocytes, which act as a cellular translation system, and the supernatants tested for the presence of the desired protein.

2. Synthesis of complementary DNA (cDNA).   Once the appropriate mRNA has been isolated, it is possible to synthesize a DNA molecule which is complementary to the message (cDNA). This can be achieved *in vitro* by the use of a retroviral enzyme known as reverse transcriptase (RT). Retroviruses are RNA-containing viruses which replicate inside a host cell by first synthesizing a DNA copy of their own RNA, using RT which is encoded within the viral genome. The cDNA produced on the mRNA template is single stranded and another enzyme, DNA polymerase, is used to produce a second strand complementary to the first. It is not usually possible to isolate specific mRNA without contaminating RNA coding for different proteins. Thus, when mRNA from a cell is used to prepare DNA, a cDNA 'library' results. Insertion of fragments of the cDNA library into bacterial cells will result in a large number of bacterial colonies each producing different proteins depending on the nature of the cDNA injected.

3. Insertion of DNA into cells.   In *prokaryotic cells*, most of the genetic information in bacterial cells is contained in one or more copies of a circular chromosome. In addition, many bacteria possess extrachromosomal DNA in the form of double-stranded, circular plasmids, containing very few genes. These plasmids may be exchanged between bacteria during bacterial conjugation and, since they frequently contain genes coding for antibiotic resistance, are one of the most common ways in which the property of resistance is spread between bacterial populations. Mammalian genes can be more readily inserted into bacterial plasmids rather than the larger chromosome. Pure plasmid DNA, purified from bacterial extracts by density-gradient centrifugation is sliced at specific nucleotide sequences using one of a variety of bacterial *restriction endonucleases* which results in the production of 'sticky ends' (Fig. 2.7).

Mammalian DNA similarly treated can hybridize to the 'cut' ends, and the

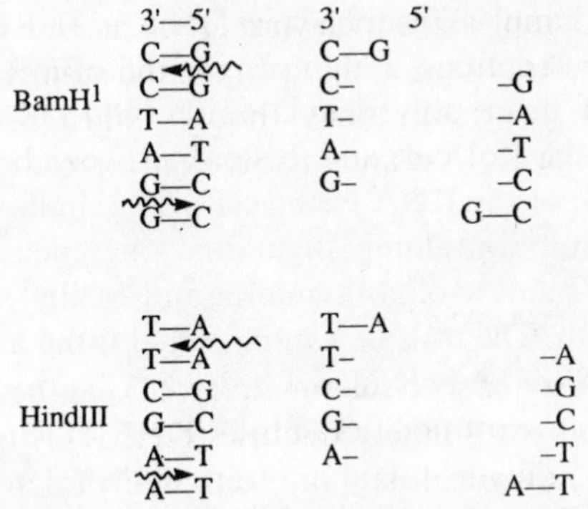

```
                3'—5'          3'      5'
                C—G            C—G
                C—G            C-           —G
      BamH¹     C—G            C-           —G
                T—A            T-           —A
                A—T            A-           —T
                G—C            G-           —C
                G—C                         G—C


                T—A            T—A
                T—A            T-           —A
                C—G            C-           —G
      HindIII   G—C            G-           —C
                A—T            A-           —T
                A—T                         A—T
```

Fig. 2.7 Action of restriction endonucleases. Several restriction endonucleases cleave DNA in such a way that they leave 'sticky ends' which can anneal to complementary sequences of DNA. Two examples shown here are the enzymes Bam H¹, from *Bacillus amyloliquefaciens* H and Hin dIII from *Haemophilus influenzae* Rd.

enzyme DNA ligase is used to 'stitch' the ends together. Plasmid DNA, containing the mammalian gene, is taken up by bacteria under appropriate culture conditions and can be monitored if the plasmid also contains an antibiotic resistance gene. The bacteria being 'transformed' do not possess the antibiotic resistance gene so that, after transformation, only those bacteria which have taken up the plasmid, will grow in a medium containing that antibiotic. Expression of the mammalian gene in *E. coli* is ensured by the insertion of prokaryotic DNA sequences known as *expression vectors* which control the expression of the gene, i.e. switch the gene on and ensure that transcription starts and stops at the appropriate place. *E. coli* 'transformants' produced in this way can be cultured in great quantities and large amounts of the lymphokine recovered from lysates of the bacteria.

The use of *eukaryotic cells* for the expression of cDNA has generally lagged behind that of prokaryotic cells for a number of reasons. For example, there is no eukaryotic equivalent of the bacterial plasmid and expression vectors are more readily available in bacterial systems. However, where glycosylation of a molecule is important for its activity *in vivo*, eukaryotic cells are essential although it is not always certain that the extent and nature of glycosylation will be the same as in the homologous cells. Mammalian cells can be readily infected with whole viruses such as SV 40 because they already carry receptor sites or they can be 'transfected' with viral DNA in a process akin to bacterial 'transformation'. Thus, viral DNA can be used as a vector for mammalian DNA which can be inserted into it through appropriate use of restriction enzymes in a manner analogous to bacterial systems. Expression vectors are not necessary since the virus already carries within its genome the information required to trigger off its own replication. One point which must be considered though is the possible contamination of the lymphokine with viral DNA or even whole virions and this may have important restrictions on the safety of the molecule which is produced. This problem is not insurmountable, though, since adequate treatment of products with DNAse or RNAse and quality-control testing for infective virions are feasible.

Amplification of gene expression

Recombinant genes inserted into mammalian cells can be amplified by making use of the gene for dihydrofolate reductase (DHFR) (Fig. 2.8). DHFR is an enzyme which reduces dihydrofolate into tetrahydrofolate, an essential step in the production of purines and pyrimidines and hence for cell growth. DHFR is inhibited by methotrexate, a drug which is active at concentrations of 10^{-9}M. Some cells can become adapted to methotrexate if they are incubated initially in very low concentrations, followed by a stepwise increase in concentration. The reason for adaptation to growth in methotrexate seems to be due to a gene dosage effect: the number of genes for DHFR is amplified some 50 to 1000-fold so that cells are able to overcome the methotrexate block. This property of gene amplification can be utilized to amplify any gene whose product is of interest because, when the gene for DHFR is amplified, other genes on the same DNA molecule are simultaneously amplified. Therefore, if a lymphokine gene such as that coding for IFN-γ is inserted into viral DNA alongside the DHFR gene, and this viral DNA is used to transfect mammalian cells in culture, the addition of methotrexate to the culture causes co-amplification of both genes so that the production of IFN-γ itself shows a corresponding increase.

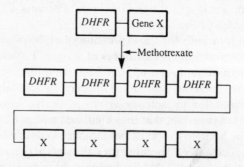

Fig. 2.8 Gene amplification. The expression of a gene can be amplified if the gene is inserted into the target cell together with a gene coding for dihydrofolate reductase (DHFR). DHFR catalyses the reduction of dihydrofolate into tetrahydrofolate. In the presence of methotrexate, a folic acid antagonist, the gene coding for DHFR is amplified, sometimes several hundredfold. Any genes close to that for DHFR (such as gene X) are also amplified.

Purification of lymphokines

Lymphokines must be purified significantly before these products can be used for research or pharmaceutical purposes. The principal contaminants will, of course, depend on the source of the molecule and this will also determine the purification procedures which can be utilized. In bacteria, the major problem is the contamination of the lymphokine with endotoxin which is pyrogenic and can sometimes result in endotoxic shock. Where the lymphokine has been produced by stimulation of lymphocytes, a host of other lymphokines are also induced which may, depending on the technique, also be contaminated by stimulatory factors such as PHA and PMA. The use of cell lines which are known to produce a particular lymphokine may be less of a problem in this respect although sensitive detection methods may later reveal that more than one lymphokine was in fact produced. Some assay systems may also detect more than one lymphokine since these frequently have an overlapping spectrum of activities. Many constitutive cell lines also present a hazard if they are derived from malignant cells such as T-cell leukaemias. There is always the danger of the presence of oncogenic, i.e. cancer-producing, viruses being also produced by such cell lines and anybody who is culturing, in particular, cell lines derived from human tumours of any kind should respect this danger and take steps to prevent and contain infection of themselves and the environment.

Ideally, any purification procedures should be sufficiently extensive as to provide preparations which would give unequivocal results (or could be safely administered to patients) but this must also inevitably result in loss of yield. PHA can be removed on affinity columns of immobilized red cells to which these lectins bind. Otherwise, the usual biochemical techniques for purifying proteins are available, including salt fractionation, ion-exchange chromatography, molecular sieve, polyacrylamide gel electrophoresis using sodium dodecyl sulphate (SDS-PAGE) and high-performance liquid chromatography (HPLC).

Immunoaffinity chromatography. This is the most commonly employed method for purification of lymphokines. It is a technique which relies on the ability of immobilized antibody to remove a protein from a mixture. Sepharose particles are 'activated' by treatment with cyanogen bromide so that they will readily take up proteins. Thus, specific antibodies to an individual lymphokine can be used to coat the surface of CNBr-activated Sepharose and a column of particles used to remove the specific protein from a 'soup' which is passed through it. The lymphokine can later be freed from its antigen–antibody complex by lowering the pH of the column (Fig. 2.9). Such a technique gave the first highly purified sample of IFN-α from virus-treated human leukocytes. The characteristics of the antibody are important here. For example, a high-affinity antibody will 'remove' a high percentage of the required protein and give a high purity. However, if the affinity is too high then the pH required to free the protein may be so low as to denature it significantly. It might be politic to choose a lower affinity antibody,

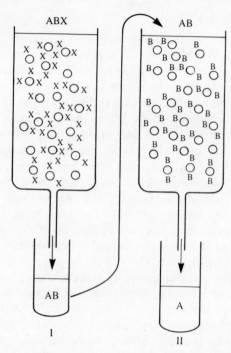

Fig. 2.9 Affinity chromatography. Purification of a lymphokine by affinity chromatography. Column I contains cyanogen bromide-activated Sepharose beads coated with a monoclonal antibody to the protein X. When the mixture containing A, B and X (ABX) is applied to the column, X binds to the immobilized antibody and A and B (AB) are eluted. Column II contains immobilized anti-B so that pure A is eluted. X and B can be recovered from the column by reducing the pH to 2.5.

and obtain a lower yield of a protein with a high activity. Alternatively, a negative selection technique might be considered whereby affinity columns are used to remove everything but the lymphokine required, although this will be more time-consuming and expensive in terms of monoclonal antibodies.

If a specific antibody is not available, lymphokines have to be purified by using particular biophysical properties. For example, IL-2 can be obtained from the supernatants of the cell line MLA-144 by concentrating the supernatants against methyl cellulose preparations, and precipitating with saturated ammonium sulphate, this process being preceded and succeeded by extensive dialysis against phosphate-buffered saline. Many lymphokines may be sequentially purified from tissue culture media or the lysates of bacteria such as *E. coli* by the use of familiar biochemical techniques, for example, a preliminary purification with ammonium sulphate followed by ion-exchange chromatography or gel filtration.

To illustrate the type of approach which may be taken, the isolation of mouse IL-3 from supernatants of the mouse myelomonocytic cell line WEHI-3B and of recombinant IL-3 from *E. coli* are outlined in Fig. 2.10.

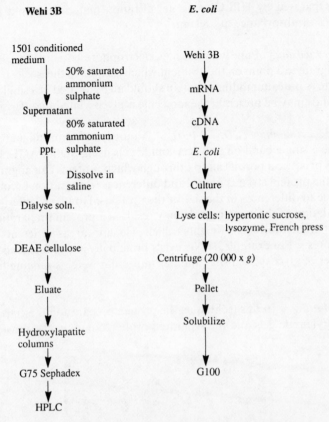

Fig. 2.10 Purification of IL-3 from WEHI-3B and *E. coli*. This demonstrates actual procedures previously used to purify native IL-3 from a mammalian cell line and recombinant IL-3 from *E. coli*. See Clark-Lewis *et al.* (1986), Ihle *et al.* (1982) and Fung *et al.* (1984).

Quality control

It is important with any purification procedure to sample the product at various stages of the purification and analyse its purity and biological activity by an appropriate assay system – a highly purified lymphokine is not much use if, somewhere along the line, the molecule has been rendered inactive by part of the isolation procedures. Chapter 3 gives an account of some general and more specific assay procedures. The purity of the sample can be ascertained by standard procedures such as those listed below.

High-performance liquid chromatography (HPLC). The use of pressure pumps to force a liquid phase over a stationary phase packed into a small stainless-steel column provides a rapid chromatographic system of high resolution. Pure proteins separated by HPLC using gel filtration materials should produce a single peak of absorbance at 280 nm.

Isoelectric focusing.   Pure lymphokines electrophoresed across a pH gradient should migrate to a point on the gradient which is equal to the isoelectric point of the protein. A pure, unmodified protein should all be located in a single band but several bands may be present if the molecule is glycosylated to differing degrees.

Sodium dodecyl sulphate (SDS–PAGE).   A pure lymphokine might be expected to produce a single band on polyacrylamide gels using SDS–PAGE. Polyacrylamide gels produce a porous matrix through which proteins can migrate. If SDS is added, the protein strands unfold and differences in migration become almost entirely due to differences in the size of the proteins. However, differing degrees of glycosylation of the same peptide may result in a protein preparation having several different molecular weights which will appear as different bands on electrophoresis. For example, IFN-γ exists principally in two forms according to the number of glycosylated sites and has molecular weights ranging from 20 to 25 kDa.

Western blotting.   In this technique, the protein preparation is electrophoresed on polyacrylamide gels and the separated protein components transferred to a

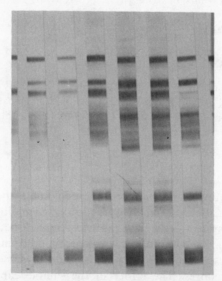

Fig. 2.11 Western blotting. Proteins separated by SDS–PAGE are blotted onto nitrocellulose filters and probed with a specific antibody. The latter is visualized by an enzyme-labelled anti-immunoglobulin. The enzyme is one which converts a colourless compound into an insoluble coloured product. (Photograph courtesy of R. Abbott, Public Health Laboratory, Withington Hospital.)

nitrocellulose filter by blotting. The filter is then incubated with a specific antibody to the lymphokine and this is then localized with an anti-immunoglobulin labelled with a radiolabel or an enzyme which can produce a coloured product (Fig. 2.11). If a specific antibody is used, the number of bands produced will indicate the number of naturally occurring forms of the polypeptide, taking account of differing degrees of glycosylation. Since the original SDS–PAGE will separate according to size, gross differences in labelled products may indicate either cleavage products retaining epitope specificity, or the presence of the lymphokine in oligomeric forms. Recombinant products produced in bacteria will not be glycosylated and should ideally produce single bands.

Where the lymphokine is to be injected either for research or for pharmaceutical purposes, it is essential to test for the presence of pyrogen. This can be achieved by careful monitoring of the temperature of injected laboratory animals. The procedure outlined above for the purification of recombinant IL-3 from *E. coli* is said to give < 2 ng lipopolysaccharide/ml of IL-3.

Summary

This chapter has dealt with the general methods which are currently available for the production of lymphokines and interleukins. Many methods discussed here are suitable only when extensive purity is not required or especially when they are not required for pharmaceutical purposes. Most large-scale preparation of these proteins is nowadays achieved by recombinant DNA technology using plasmid vectors in *E. coli*. More recently, some human lymphokines are being produced by insertion of the gene into other mammalian cell lines using virus vectors. These lymphokines have the advantage of being glycosylated although the yield of the lymphokine is generally lower. Finally, purification and assessment of purity of the preparation have also been discussed. Chapter 3 will deal with methods which are available for the biochemical characterization and assay of these molecules.

References

Brown, T. A. (1986). *Gene Cloning: An Introduction*, London, Van Nostrand Reinhold.

Butler, M. (1987). *Animal Cell Technology: Principles and Products*, OUP Biotechnology Series. Milton Keynes, Open University Press.

Clark-Lewis, I., Aebersold, R., Zilterner, H. *et al.* (1986). 'Automated chemical synthesis of a protein growth factor for haemopoietic cell, interleukin 3', *Science*, **231**, p. 134.

Clemens, M. J., Morris, A. A. and Gearing, A. J. H. (1987). *Lymphokines and Interferons. A Practical Approach*. Oxford, IRL Press.

Dumonde, D. C., Wolstencroft, R. A., Panayi, G. S. *et al.* (1969). 'Lymphokines: non-antibody mediators of cellular immunity generated by lymphocyte activation', *Nature (London)*, **224**, p. 38.

Fung, M. C., Hapel, A. J., Ymer, S. *et al.* (1984). 'Molecular cloning of cDNA for murine interleukin-3', *Nature*, **307**, p. 233.

Ihle, J. N., Keller, J., Henderson, L. *et al.* (1982). 'Procedure for the purification of IL-3 to homogeneity', *J. Immunol.* **129**, p. 2431.

Iscove, N. and Schreier, M. H. (1979). 'Clonal growth of cells in semisolid or viscous medium' in *Immunological Methods*, Eds Lefkovitz, I. and Pernis, B. London Academic Press.

Kohler, G. (1979). 'Soft agar cloning of lymphoid tumor lines: detection of hybrid clones with anti-SRBC activity' in *Immunological Methods*, Eds Lefkovitz, I. and Pernis, B. London, Academic Press.

Lefkovitz, I. (1979). 'Limiting dilution analysis' in *Immunological Methods*, Eds Lefkovitz, I. and Pernis, B. London, Academic Press.

Morgan, D. A., Ruscetti, F. W. and Gallo, R. (1976). 'Selective *in vitro* growth of T lymphocytes from normal human bone marrow', *Science*, **193**, p. 1007.

Mossman, T. R. and Coffman, R. L. (1987). 'Two types of mouse helper T cell clone – implications for immune regulation', *Immunology Today*, **8**, p. 223.

Sandvig, S., Laskay, T., Andersson, J. *et al.* (1987). 'Gamma interferon is produced by CD3$^+$ and CD3$^-$ lymphocytes', *Immunol. Rev.*, **97**, p. 51.

Taussig, M. T. (1985). *T Cell Hybridomas*, Boca Raton, Florida, CRC Press.

Walker, J. M. and Gingold, E. B. (1988). *Molecular Biology and Biotechnology*. Cambridge, Royal Society of Chemistry.

Winnaker, E.-L. (1987). *From Genes to Clones*, W. Germany, VCH Press.

Wrigglesworth, J. M. (1983). *Biochemical Research Techniques: A Practical Introduction*. Chichester, John Wiley.

3

Biochemical Characterization of Lymphokines

Introduction

The previous chapter discussed the relative merits of different methods for producing and purifying proteins. Once sufficient pure protein has been obtained by whatever means, several approaches to the biochemical characterization of the molecule may be adopted. In addition, the purified protein, and monoclonal antibodies prepared against it, can be used to analyse the quantity, distribution, and biochemical nature of lymphokine receptors on the surface of lymphokine-sensitive target cells. This information is needed when studying the mode of action of lymphokines and may also be useful therapeutically, perhaps for preventing potentially harmful effects of molecules such as tumour necrosis factor (TNF). In this chapter, the different approaches to the study of lymphokines and their receptors will be discussed. The methods for locating lymphokine genes will also be outlined since a greater understanding of the interaction and regulation of lymphokine genes, and of diseases characterized by aberrant lymphokine production, is dependent on knowledge of their precise chromosomal location. One such example is the myelodysplastic syndrome where low levels of blood leukocytes can be linked to deletions of chromosome 5, in the region of several lymphokine genes, including interleukin-3 (IL-3), a haemopoietic growth factor.

Finally, extensive purification and characterization of a molecule is little use unless there are ways of proving, firstly that the right lymphokine has been obtained and secondly, that it is still active. In this chapter, several methods for assaying the quantity and activity of lymphokines will be discussed. The overlapping nature of lymphokine-mediated activities makes the choice of assay for individual lymphokines particularly difficult.

Biochemical characterization

In the early days of lymphokine research many of the biochemical techniques for analysing biologically active 'factors' in the supernatants of stimulated lymphocytes were laborious and time-consuming. In the first instance it was necessary to establish the molecular nature of the factor and this was usually approached by studying the effects of adding proteases or neuraminidase to the lymphokine 'soup' in order to establish the protein or glycoprotein nature of the molecules. Nowadays, it is accepted that lymphokines or interleukins are proteins and indeed they are defined as such. Various procedures can be used to determine the physical properties of the molecule including the molecular weight, the number of polypeptide chains making up the protein, the degree of polymerization of the protein *in vivo* and its three-dimensional structure. Most important, though, is to determine the amino acid sequence, and this can be achieved by analysis of the protein itself or of a cDNA coding for the protein.

PHYSICAL PROPERTIES

An estimate of the molecular weight of the lymphokine can be made by gel filtration on Sephadex. Columns of Sephadex of different pore sizes can be used to determine the size range of the molecule initially by finding the smallest pore size in which it is retained. The volume of buffer then required to elute the lymphokine from that column can be compared with the buffer volumes needed to elute a range of proteins of different sizes (Fig. 3.1) and this provides a rough estimate of its molecular weight.

Electrophoresis of the protein on polyacrylamide gels has provided much information on the physical properties of lymphokines and interleukins. The

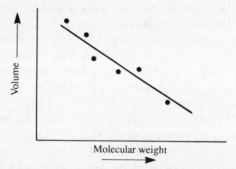

Fig. 3.1 Estimation of molecular weight by gel filtration. A Sephadex column can be calibrated by measuring the volume required to elute a protein of known molecular weight. If several proteins are used a graph can be plotted of volume against molecular weight. This graph can be used to estimate the molecular weight of an unknown protein from its elution volume.

technique can be used to determine the molecular weight of a protein and differences between the figure obtained with native and recombinant protein produced in bacteria will give an indication of the degree of polymerization and glycosylation of the naturally occurring molecule. Polyacrylamide gels are particularly useful for electrophoresis as they are stable in a wide range of buffers, and can be easily produced with different pore sizes by varying the concentration of the monomer. In addition, they are transparent and do not absorb UV light so that proteins, which absorb maximally at 280 nm can be readily located using a UV lamp. A rapid separation can be achieved and, following electrophoresis, the gels can be incubated with a protein stain, such as Coumassie brilliant blue R250 or with a periodic acid–Schiff's stain for glycoproteins. A stained gel can be scanned with a densitometer which measures the density of colour (Fig. 3.2).

A variation of polyacrylamide gel electrophoresis (PAGE), commonly used to separate proteins because it gives high resolution of protein bands, includes sodium dodecyl sulphate (SDS) and 2-mercaptoethanol (2ME) in the protein mixture. SDS is a powerful detergent which dissolves protein aggregates linked by hydrophobic interactions. The combination of 2ME, a reducing agent and SDS with the protein, followed by brief boiling, results in the denaturation of the protein to its individual polypeptide chains. Under these conditions, all proteins have a similar charge so that the speed of migration is entirely dependent on the size of the molecule, smaller proteins being the most mobile. The molecular weight can be ascertained by comparison with a standard gel separation of a mixture of proteins of known molecular weights. Comparison between

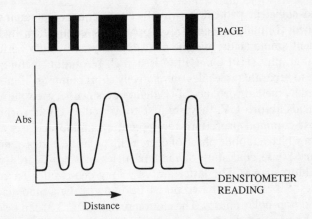

Fig. 3.2 Polyacrylamide gel electrophoresis. In an electric field, proteins will migrate through the pores of a polyacrylamide gel. In the presence of SDS the distance travelled is inversely related to the size of the protein. If the gel is stained, for example with Coumassie blue, after the separation is completed, the gel can be scanned in a densitometer, to yield a series of peaks and troughs depending on the presence and concentration of the protein.

SDS–PAGE and PAGE under non-reducing conditions may give some indication of the degree of polymerization of the molecule or the number of polypeptide chains which make up the active protein. Having said this, the lymphokines and interleukins, so far studied, consist of a single polypeptide chain, although these may occasionally occur as dimers. SDS–PAGE techniques can also be used preparatively and proteins eluted from slices of the unstained gel. The recovered proteins can be 'renatured' if the SDS is removed by extensive dialysis or by ion-exchange chromatography.

In addition to PAGE, other biochemical techniques such as isoelectric focusing can be used both analytically and preparatively. In isoelectric focusing, the molecule is electrophoresed across a pH gradient, coming to rest at the region of the gradient corresponding to the isoelectric pH (pI) of the molecule. Since the pI is affected both by the amino acid composition and, if it is glycosylated, by the character of the oligosaccharides, isoelectric focusing can provide information on either. For example, a single gene codes for human IL-2 but at least two molecules can be separated by this technique. One of these molecules has an acidic pI due to sialic acid residues in the carbohydrate moiety. The differing contributions of amino acid residues or glycosylation to the pI can be ascertained by comparing glycosylated and non-glycosylated forms. Carbohydrate can be chemically or enzymatically removed from glycoproteins and non-glycosylated recombinant forms can be produced in prokaryotes, or in eukaryotic cells grown in the presence of inhibitors of glycosylation, such as tunicamycin.

DETERMINATION OF PROTEIN SEQUENCES

Provided sufficient protein is available, the sequence of amino acids can be determined. Initially a sample of protein is completely hydrolysed to its constituent amino acids, and the mixture analysed by high-performance liquid chromatography (HPLC). HPLC is a high-resolution technique which uses pressure to separate molecules on relatively short columns. Eluted materials are measured by their absorbance of UV light but, since very few naturally occurring amino acids absorb UV, they are first converted to UV-absorbing derivatives. The most common procedure for separating amino acids is a reverse-phase HPLC in which a mobile phase of decreasing polarity, elutes amino acids from a stationary phase consisting of inert particles of silica coated with non-polar organochlorosilanes. The latter are very long-chain silica-based hydrophobic molecules. Separation is based on partitioning of the amino acids between the polar and non-polar phases. The elution profile (Fig. 3.3) can be compared with that of known standards under identical conditions. The quantities of each amino acid can be determined from the area of each peak, provided that an internal standard, such as L-norleucine is added to the sample prior to separation. The amino acid sequence of the protein may be determined by degrading the molecule, one residue at a time, from the end of the molecule. One such analytical method is the Edman degradation in which amino acids are

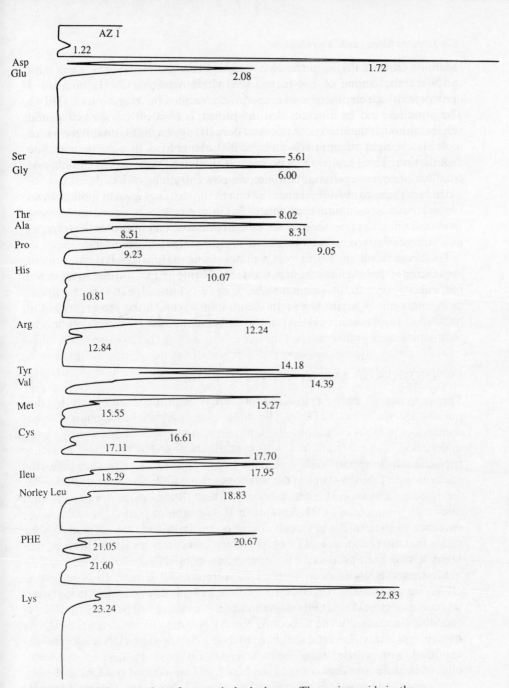

Fig. 3.3 HPLC separation of a protein hydrolysate. The amino acids in the hydrolysate were reacted with phenylisothiocyanate to form phenylthiocarbamyl derivatives. The separation was achieved on a C18 column with a gradient of aqueous buffer and acetonitrile. L-Norleu is not an amino acid found in proteins but was used as an internal standard. (Courtesy of Dr M. Butler.)

identified sequentially from the N-terminus. Phenylisothiocyanate reacts with the N-terminal amino acid to form a phenylthiohydantoin (PTH)-amino acid derivative, which can then be separated and identified by reverse-phase HPLC. The procedure can be automated if the protein is covalently bound to a solid support prior to degradation. Approximately 100 μg of a pure lymphokine with a molecular weight of approximately 15 000 are needed to achieve complete degradation. This may prove a problem if the lymphokine has been obtained from lymphocyte supernatants where the concentrations of individual lymphokines are in the pg/ml–ng/ml range although this does not present quite such an obstacle with recombinant proteins. A more recent technique, requiring a thousand times less protein, uses the Edman degradation but carries the reagents in a stream of argon to the protein which is immobilized on a film.

The sequencing of entire polypeptides using improved classical protein sequencing techniques has the disadvantage of being extremely time consuming, particularly when the protein has to be extensively purified first. It is now much more common to predict the sequence of amino acids in the protein from the nucleotide sequence in a cDNA, the latter being much more easily determined than amino acid sequences.

PREDICTION OF AMINO ACID SEQUENCES

The sequence of amino acids in a protein is determined ultimately by the nucleotide sequence in the DNA. The triplet code, in which the sequence of three nucleotides in DNA codes for a single amino acid residue, is now extremely well understood. Over 20 different amino acids are found in proteins, and the triplet(s) which specify each one have been identified. Given four different nucleotides in DNA, 64 triplet combinations are possible. Sixty-one triplets code for specific amino acids, the remaining three being 'stop' codons. If the nucleotide sequence of a cDNA is known, it is possible to predict the amino acid sequence in the protein to a high degree of accuracy. Analysis of the cDNA, rather than the chromosomal DNA, is preferred since introns are not present, the DNA having been produced by transcription of mRNA.

Messenger RNA from a lymphokine-secreting cell is used to construct a cDNA library, which takes the form of clones of transformed bacteria carrying fragments of the cDNA. Only a fraction of these clones will be carrying cDNA encoding the desired protein, because the mRNA used to construct the cDNA library represents the total cellular mRNA. The desired cDNA clones are identified with a specific probe which, in this case, is a short synthetic oligonucleotide complementary to the first 7 or 8 amino acid residues at the N-terminus of the protein, as determined by partial Edman degradation. Plasmid DNA is purified from different clones, heated to separate the two strands and incubated with the radiolabelled probe which will hybridize only to plasmid DNA containing the complementary sequence. Positive clones are amplified and the cDNA obtained by splicing the plasmid DNA with appropriate restriction enzymes (Fig. 3.4).

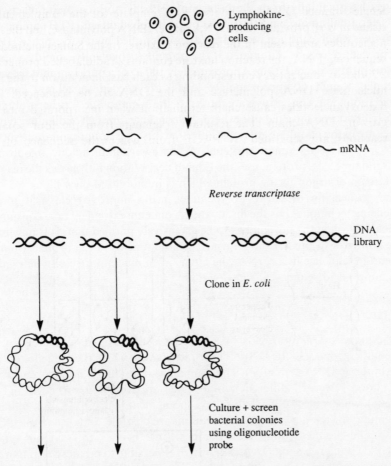

Fig. 3.4 Construction of a cDNA library. Total mRNA is extracted from cells which are secreting the desired lymphokine and transcribed into cDNA using reverse transcriptase. Fragments of cDNA are inserted into bacterial plasmids and used to transform *E. coli*. Individual bacteria are grown to produce colonies. The colonies are screened by probing the bacterial DNA with an oligonucleotide probe complementary to the N-terminal amino acid sequence of the lymphokine.

DETERMINING THE SEQUENCE OF THE cDNA

The sequence of nucleotides in the cDNA is determined by one of two methods:

(1) DNA is radiolabelled at one end of the molecule and is then chemically cleaved, in four separate reactions, under conditions which specifically cleave the DNA at each of the four nucleotides (A,T,C,G). Products of the cleavage are separated by PAGE according to size and an autoradiograph prepared. The sequence of nucleotides can be determined by relating increasing sizes of fragments to the chemical cleavage site (Fig. 3.5a).

(2) Single-stranded DNA can be used as a template for the complementary strand *in vitro* provided that a DNA primer, DNA polymerase, and the four nucleotides are present in the reaction mixture. In the Sanger method for sequencing DNA, the reaction mixture contains a radiolabelled primer and 2'3'-dideoxynucleotides corresponding to each base in addition to the four nucleotides, DNA polymerase and the DNA to be sequenced. 2'3'-dideoxynucleotides cause chain termination when incorporated into the growing DNA chain. The resultant fragments from the four separate reactions are separated by PAGE from which the sequence of the

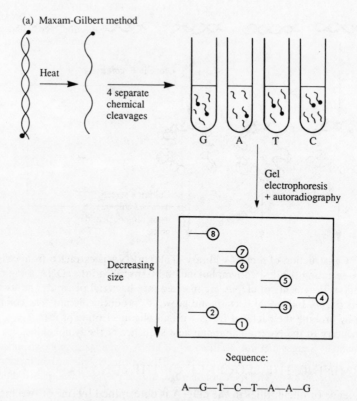

Sequence:

A—G—T—C—T—A—A—G

Fig. 3.5 DNA sequencing. (a) Maxam–Gilbert method. Radiolabelled DNA is rendered single-stranded by heating and four samples are subjected to chemical treatment which cleaves the strand at G, A, T and C nucleotide residues, respectively. The four samples are then subjected to gel electrophoresis and the electrophoretogram examined by autoradiography. The sequence can then be 'read' from the lowest molecular-weight fragments to the highest.

complementary strand (and therefore of the original strand) can be determined (Fig. 3.5b).

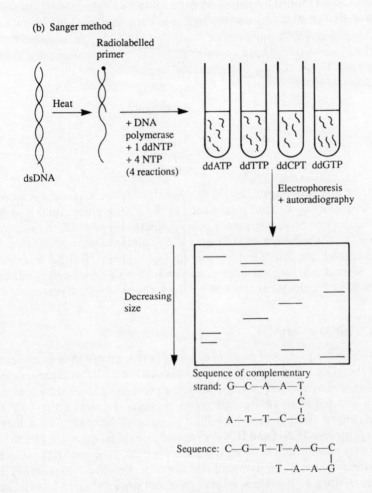

Fig 3.5 *cont.* (b) Sanger method. Radiolabelled DNA is rendered single-stranded and allowed to anneal to a short, complementary, DNA primer. This is then incubated on four separate occasions with DNA polymerase, the four nucleotides, plus a dideoxy (dd) derivative of one of the four nucleotides. Dideoxynucleotides cause chain termination when incorporated in place of its corresponding deoxynucleotide. Thus, a series of complementary DNA fragments will be synthesized representing chain terminations at the appropriate nucleotide in the sequence. The fragments are separated by electrophoresis and read as in (a). On this occasion, though, the sequence read is that of the complementary DNA strand, from which can be deduced the sequence of the actual DNA strand.

The amino acid sequence of a protein which has been determined from a cDNA sequence can never be regarded as completely accurate because an error in the identification of a single nucleotide will result in the prediction of the wrong amino acid. For example the triplet AGC specifies the amino acid serine. A single nucleotide change in each case specifies:

TGC	Cysteine
CGC	Arginine
GGC	Glycine
ATC	Isoleucine
AAC	Asparagine
ACC	Threonine
AGA	Arginine
AGG	Arginine
AGT	Serine

In addition, it is important to establish where the cDNA sequence for a protein begins since starting to read a sequence in the wrong place could lead to an entirely inaccurate protein sequence being predicted. In practice, this is not such a problem, since the N-terminal sequence of 6–7 amino acids may well have been determined and one can therefore line up this sequence with the code on the cDNA. Several years ago predicted amino acid sequences were published as having a 95% accuracy but this has been improved in recent years.

COMPUTER DATABANKS

The amino acid sequences of proteins can now be determined in days, rather than years, if the cDNA is available. This has resulted in an information explosion concerning amino acid sequences of different proteins. The information can be stored in databanks so that comparisons between the sequences of different proteins can be compared. Where high degrees of homology exist between different proteins – IFN-α and IFN-β are good examples – there is likely to be an evolutionary relationship between the genes for these proteins. Databanks have been extremely useful in lymphokine research because lymphokines have multiple activities *in vivo*. Thus, several groups of workers might be sequencing, respectively, B-cell stimulatory factor-2 (BSF2), HPGF (hybridoma plasmacytoma growth factor), and interferon-β2, only to discover that all these molecules are identical (IL-6, see Chapter 8).

Determination of structure–function relationships

The tertiary structure of a protein is very important in determining its biological activity, since folding exposes particular regions and 'hides' others. The stability of the tertiary structure is partly determined by covalent disulphide links between

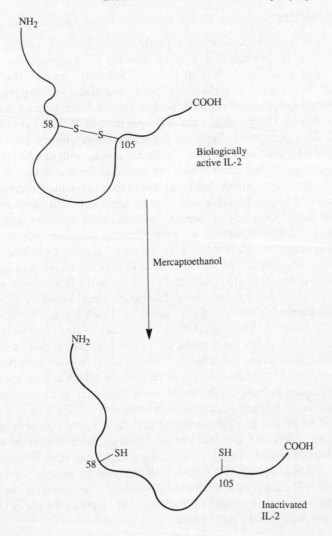

Fig. 3.6 Reduction of interleukin-2. The importance of a disulphide link to the biological activity of a protein can be assessed by looking at the activity after reduction of the molecule with mercaptoethanol. Interleukin-2 has an essential disulphide link between cysteine residues at amino acids 58 and 105. Reduction of this bridge results in total loss of activity.

cysteine residues. The importance of disulphide links can be determined by assaying the biological activity of the lymphokine following reduction and alkylation of the molecule (Fig. 3.6). The activity of human IL-2, for example, is completely lost after this treatment. Disulphide links stabilize the folding of protein, and loss of activity indicates the importance of the shape of these molecules.

AMINO ACIDS

Where there is doubt concerning a particular amino acid, and an alternative sequence can be predicted, it may be possible to synthesize the alternative protein, and assay its biological activity. Recently, murine IL-3 has been produced in a peptide synthesizer. Such machines are capable of being programmed to produce peptides with a specified amino acid sequence, by chemical means. The process of building up a peptide of the length of IL-3 takes about 2 days altogether. Such an approach offers endless opportunity for research since minor substitutions of different amino acids can be produced and in this way the amino acids which are essential for the active site(s) of the molecule (that site which binds to the receptor) can be determined by substitution. Shorter peptides can also be produced and these could prove extremely useful for studying peptides with multiple activities such as lymphokines where different parts of the molecule may subserve different activities.

An alternative to synthesizing peptides is to use the technique of *in vitro mutagenesis* whereby cDNA is altered so as to produce amino acid substitutions or deletions in the translated product. Fragments of the DNA can be removed by using a combination of restriction and ligase enzymes. Similarly, by cutting the DNA at a particular restriction site, and using DNA ligase, an oligonucleotide can also be inserted. Although there are a number of ways in which the cDNA can be altered, perhaps the method with most potential is one in which single nucleotide substitutions result in single amino acid changes in the protein. Thus the importance of that amino acid in relation to others can be ascertained. A short synthetic oligonucleotide strand, complementary to part of the cDNA, is constructed with a single nucleotide substitution (Fig. 3.7). The oligonucleotide is allowed to anneal to single-stranded cDNA and acts as a primer for DNA polymerase. Thus the oligonucleotide becomes part of a fully synthesized polynucleotide strand. The double stranded DNA can now be inserted into a plasmid and used to transfect *E. coli*. Half the progeny will contain the mutated DNA and will thus produce 'abnormal' protein. The effects of the nucleotide substitution can be examined by looking at the activity of the protein in the appropriate functional assay system.

CARBOHYDRATES

Knowledge of the amino acid sequence can give some indication of the location of carbohydrate residues in a glycoprotein. Carbohydrates are joined to a single amino acid residue by one of two linkages: *O-glycosidic* links in which the carbohydrate is attached via the hydroxyl groups of serine, threonine, hydroxylysine or hydroxyproline, whereas *N-glycosidic* links join the carbohydrate to asparagine via the amide nitrogen when asparagine is part of the sequence Asn–X–Ser/Thre in which X can be any residue except proline or aspartic acid. Thus potential N-glycosylation sites can be predicted with a higher degree of

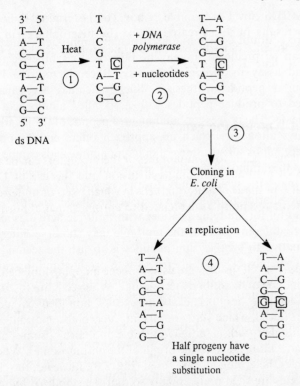

Fig. 3.7 *In vitro* mutagenesis. Double-stranded DNA is heated to separate the two strands (1) and a single strand is allowed to anneal to a short oligonucleotide primer containing a single nucleotide substitution. In the presence of DNA polymerase and the four nucleotides, a complementary strand is synthesized with a single base substitution (2). The double-stranded DNA is inserted into bacteria (3) so that at DNA replication half the progeny of the bacteria will contain this altered DNA (4). Since the DNA will now code for a protein with a single amino acid substitution, the importance of the original amino acid to the activity of the protein can be gauged.

accuracy than O-glycosylation sites since these triplet sequences occur less frequently than the single amino acid residue.

The role of glycosylation in lymphokine biochemistry is only poorly understood, but some conclusions can be made by comparing the activities of the glycosylated and non-glycosylated forms. In addition, some generalizations can be made concerning the role of glycosylation as it applies to non-lymphokine proteins. The removal of carbohydrate has little effect on the biological activity of lymphokines generally, and recombinant proteins produced in prokaryotes are as active as eukaryotic forms. Glycosylation does, however, affect the half-life of many proteins including some lymphokines, possibly by conferring resistance to proteolysis. The presence of carbohydrate may also affect the distribution of proteins. For example, removal of the terminal sialic acid residues from IFN-γ results in its increased uptake by macrophages in the liver. In addition, the presence of carbohydrate in some proteins is related to the folding of the protein chain at that site.

Location of lymphokine genes

Mapping of genes coding for lymphokines or their receptors can be achieved by a combination of methods including cell fusion and the use of DNA probes. Studies can also be made of abnormal cells in which over- or under-expression of a lymphokine or receptor can be related to chromosomal abnormalities.

CELL FUSION

The techniques for cell fusion were used for gene mapping long before they were adapted for monoclonal antibody technology. When cells are fused in syngeneic (genetically identical) or allogeneic (same species, non-identical) combinations, the hybrid produced, which starts out having a chromosome content four times the haploid number (4n), is initially unstable and chromosomes are shed, in a random fashion with regard to the origin of the chromosomes. When cells from different species (heterologous) are fused (Fig. 3.8), however, the chromosomes from one species are shed preferentially so that the stabilized hybrid may have almost a full component from one species but only one or two chromosomes from the second species. For some unspecified reason, when human and murine cells are fused, human chromosomes are preferentially shed. Normal diploid human and mouse cells have 46 and 40 chromosomes, respectively. Man/mouse hybrids, when stabilized, have between 41 and 55 chromosomes, including the entire complement of mouse chromosomes. Thus, it is not uncommon to end up with a man/mouse hybrid containing only one human chromosome which can be identified by features such as the size and shape of the chromosome, the position of the centromere, and the banding pattern when the chromosomes are stained by the Giemsa technique (G-bands). If the hybrid expresses any 'human' protein, it must be because that gene is located on the one remaining human chromosome. The production of a range of hybrids carrying different human chromosomes has allowed many proteins to be mapped to a particular chromosome. Similarly, in some chromosal abnormalities, there may be complete or partial deletion of a chromosome. Absence of a protein in that individual can be related to the loss of that chromosome which is therefore most likely to be the site of that particular gene. In addition, extra chromosomes can often be related to excess production of proteins. For example, in Down's syndrome there is trisomy of chromosome 21. Cells from these individuals have high numbers of the receptor for IFN-α and IFN-β.

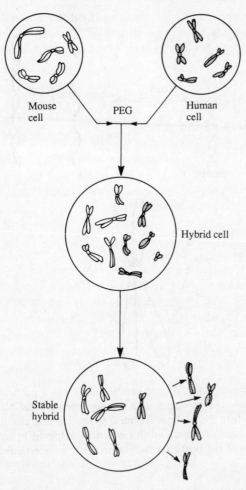

Fig. 3.8 Mapping lymphokine genes. The fusion of a mouse cell with a human cell, using polyethyleneglycol (PEG) results in the production of an unstable hybrid. This hybrid preferentially sheds human chromosomes and eventually stabilizes with perhaps a single human chromosome. If the cell expresses a human protein, it must be encoded by that chromosome.

IN SITU HYBRIDIZATION

DNA hybridization depends on the annealing of single-stranded DNA to another DNA strand if there is sufficient complementarity between the two strands. DNA can be rendered single-stranded if the hydrogen bonding between the two strands is broken down by heat or extremes of pH (Fig. 3.9). The amount of annealling can be measured if one strand is radiolabelled, for example with ^{32}P.

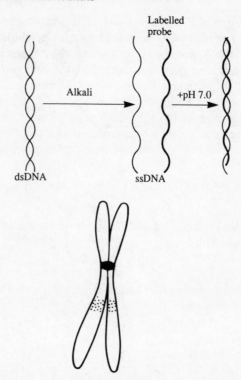

Fig. 3.9 *In situ* hybridization. A gene can be mapped to a particular chromosome by probing metaphase chromosomes with a complementary radiolabelled DNA probe. However, before the probe will anneal to the relevant chromosome, the DNA must be rendered single-stranded and this is usually achieved by treatment with alkali. The presence of the probe on the chromosome is ascertained by autoradiography.

A radioactively labelled DNA probe is a piece of DNA complementary to one of the strands specifying a particular gene. It can be used to locate the gene on metaphase chromosomes either within the cell itself or within a man/mouse hybrid cell. In practice, the cells are treated with 50% formamide, which lowers the melting temperature of the DNA, and heated to 67–70°C for 1–2 min. The radiolabelled probe is then incubated with the cell. The location of the probe, which anneals to its complementary sequence on one of the chromosomes, can be detected by autoradiography.

Lymphokine receptors

A great deal of information is now available concerning the amino acid sequences of lymphokines, and the recent developments in the techniques of computer modelling make it seem likely that the secondary and tertiary structures will soon be predictable. With the powerful techniques of recombinant DNA technology, DNA molecules containing the information required to synthesize the protein have been constructed and in many instances the genes have been mapped to particular chromosomes. In contrast, relatively little is known about the receptor molecules with which these proteins interact at the membranes of the target cells. Only one such receptor molecule, the human IL-2 receptor, has been characterized to a significant extent although the chromosomal location of several human lymphokine receptor genes have been located.

BIOCHEMICAL CHARACTERIZATION OF MEMBRANE RECEPTORS

The binding of a ligand to a receptor is an equilibrium reaction which follows the Law of Mass Action. Thus:

$$L + R \leftrightarrow LR$$

where L is the ligand (lymphokine) and R is the receptor. The rate, R^1, of the forward reaction is proportional to the concentrations of the reactants. Thus:

$$R^1 = k_a \, [L][R]$$

and the rate, R^2, of the backward reaction:

$$R^2 = k_d \, [LR]$$

where k_a and k_d are the rate constants for association and dissociation, respectively. At equilibrium, $R^1 = R^2$. Therefore:

$$k_a \, [L][R] = k_d \, [LR]$$

The ratio of the rate constants for association and dissociation is:

$$\frac{k_a}{k_d} = K_a = \frac{[LR]}{[L][R]}$$

The affinity constant K_a has dimensions of l/mole. In practice, the dissociation constant, K_d, which is the reciprocal of the affinity constant, is usually quoted. K_d is therefore equal to the concentration of ligand which results in 50% of the binding sites being occupied. Thus if K_d is low, e.g. 10^{-12} M, the affinity of the receptors is very high since the ligand need only be present at a concentration of 10^{-12} M, in order to achieve 50% saturation of the receptors.

In attempts to estimate the number and affinity of specific receptor molecules on the surface of cells, two approaches have been adopted. The first, and most common, is to measure the binding of radiolabelled ligand to the surface of cells. Pure lymphokine is radiolabelled, usually by iodination with ^{125}I, and a given number of target cells are incubated with lymphokine solutions of increasing concentrations. It is a good idea to choose as a target, cells which are very

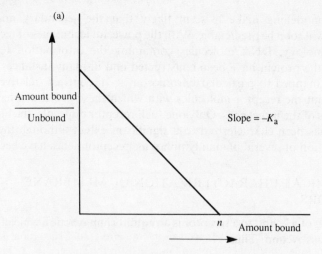

Affinity constant, $K_a = 1/K_d$; n = number of binding sites

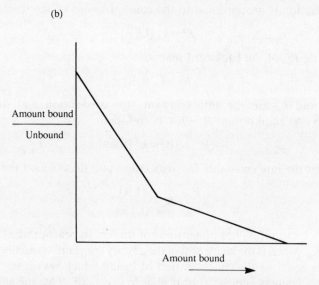

Fig. 3.10 Lymphokine receptors.
(a) Scatchard plots can be used to estimate the number of binding sites on a cell and the affinity constant of these receptors. Cells are incubated with varying concentrations of radiolabelled lymphokine and the amount of label bound is measured. The slope of the Scatchard is used to calculate the affinity constant, K_a, and the intercept on the X-axis gives the number of binding sites.
(b) If a Scatchard plot fails to give a straight line, it indicates receptors with different binding affinities. In the plot shown there is a single inflection, indicative of two different affinities.

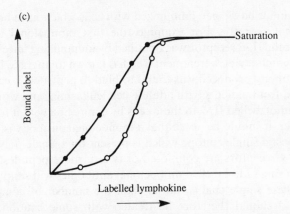

Fig. 3.10 *cont.* (c) If the binding of a radiolabelled lymphokine is inhibited by another lymphokine it is possible that they bind to the same receptor. The graph shows the binding of radiolabelled lymphokine to target cells in the absence (●) and in the presence (○) of a fixed amount of a second lymphokine which binds to the same receptor.

sensitive to the activity of that lymphokine, since, not only are these cells more likely to have higher numbers of receptors, but the degree of binding at different concentrations can also be compared with dose–response curves for biological activity. After incubation of the cells with radiolabelled lymphokine, the cells are washed extensively to remove non-bound lymphokine and the radioactivity counted. The figures can be represented in a Scatchard plot (Fig. 3.10a) where the slope of the line is $- K_a$ and the point at which this line crosses the X-axis, n, gives the number of available binding sites. A Scatchard plot also gives an indication of the variability of binding sites because a straight line is obtained only if all the binding sites are homogeneous. If the Scatchard plot is not a straight line (Fig. 3.10b), this means that the receptors are not homogeneous, the number of inflections indicating the number of different receptors of different affinity. A plot of bound radiolabel against increasing lymphokine concentration will usually reveal a typical binding curve showing saturation at high concentrations of ligand. The binding should be inhibited by incorporation of a certain amount of 'cold' lymphokine into the reaction mixture (Fig. 3.10c). Similarly, if two molecules share the same receptor, the binding of one will be inhibited in the presence of the other. Examples of this phenomenon including TNF-α and TNF-β, IL-1α and IL-1β, and IFN-α and IFN-β. All of these pairs of lymphokines are characterized by a high degree of sequence homology indicating evolution in each case from the same ancestral gene.

The second approach to quantifying cell surface receptors has been to obtain monoclonal antibodies to epitopes on such receptors. A radiolabelled monoclonal antibody can then be treated as if it were the lymphokine and Scatchard plots prepared. In order to obtain monoclonal antibodies to cell surface receptors, animals have been immunized with cells which have been induced to synthesize that receptor. For example, the first monoclonal antibody with specificity for the IL-2 receptor was obtained by immunizing mice with mitogen-activated T-lymphocytes, a treatment which is known to upgrade IL-2R on these cells. The antibody produced was found to bind to activated T-cells, leukaemic cells obtained from patients with adult T-cell leukaemia, and would inhibit the binding of radiolabelled IL-2 to these cells by competing with it for the receptor sites. However, it should be noted that a monoclonal antibody is, by definition, directed against a single epitope which is present on a single polypeptide chain whereas many receptors are composed of two or more peptides. Thus, results obtained by using radiolabelled monoclonal antibodies will simply measure the number of these single chains, rather than the number of complete receptor molecules and should therefore be treated with some caution. Monoclonal antibodies, however, are extremely useful when trying to characterize the cell surface receptor. The membranes of target cells, pre-incubated with specific radiolabelled antibodies, can be solubilized with detergent, and the membrane proteins obtained subjected to SDS–PAGE. The protein bands can be transferred by blotting onto a nitrocellulose filter and the radiolabelled band detected by autoradiography. By comparing the gel with known standards, the size of the receptor/antibody complex can be ascertained and, knowing the molecular weight of the antibody (from its class) an estimate of the size of the receptor made. The molecular characterization of the receptor can be approached in the same way as the lymphokine. The receptor can be obtained by removing the bound antibody by gel filtration at low pH, or by cloning the cDNA gene, prepared from mRNA obtained from cells in which the expression of the receptor has been induced.

Lymphokine assay

Sensitive and accurate lymphokine assays are essential in many fields of immunological and biotechnological research as well as being essential for monitoring purification procedures. The chosen assay should be discriminatory so that as far as possible only the lymphokine in question is being measured. Lymphokine assays may be used, for example, to determine the products of T-cell hybridomas, or of helper or cytotoxic T-cell clones. Similarly, determining the optimum culture conditions so as to maximize lymphokine products of mammalian or prokaryotic cells necessitates reliable assay systems which are quick and easy to perform. In medicine and biomedical research, one might wish to assay a particular lymphokine in order to assess a patient's immune deficit: patients with AIDS, for example, are deficient particularly in IL-2 and any attempts to restore this deficit will require extremely sensitive assays. In summary, therefore, assays for lymphokines should, ideally, be:

- Sensitive – since most lymphokines are active in the ng–pg/ml range
- Specific – in order to detect a single lymphokine in a mixture and in a variety of different backgrounds such as tissue culture media or body fluids, without first having to purify the protein
- Reproducible – to enable results from long-term experiments to be meaningful
- Inexpensive – for obvious reasons
- Quick and easy to perform

Assay methods for lymphokines and interleukins fall into one of two major categories. First, they can be assayed by the use of tests for a particular function. An example of this might be the assay of interferons by measuring the ability of these molecules to protect cells against viral infection. Interleukin-2 can be measured by its ability to support the growth of lectin-stimulated lymphocytes. These methods fall into the more general category of bioassay and can be extremely sensitive, although like many bioassays they are prone to the type of variability which is fundamentally inherent in all biological systems. Another problem associated with the use of bioassay in lymphokine research is the fact that it is often difficult to find a bioassay which is exclusive to an individual lymphokine. For this reason, many assays are said to be 'promiscuous' in that they may be measuring three or four different molecules. One example is the thymocyte co-proliferation assay (see Chapter 4) which measures IL-1, IL-2 and IL-6. The full extent of this problem has only recently been appreciated. Nonetheless, if one wishes to look at the effects of *in vitro* mutagenesis, or indeed any other chemical manipulation of the protein involved, it is absolutely necessary to use a functional assay.

Where functional aspects are not important, for example when the aim is to measure the amount of a lymphokine produced under varying growth conditions in order to maximize a product, immunoassay is used. Immunoassays involve the use of antibodies specific to an epitope which is, ideally, exclusive to a particular lymphokine. Since the assay is dependent on the possession of an antibody, the specificity of the assay relies on the specificity of that antibody. In order to improve the sensitivity of the assay, and also for reasons of economy, the antibody should have a high affinity (low K_d). Fortunately, it is now possible routinely to produce monoclonal antibodies to any desired epitope, even if the protein containing the epitope is not available in pure form. This is made possible by immunizing mice and isolating individual clones of antibody-producing cells. Clones found to be producing antibody are tested, and selected so that only those producing high-affinity antibodies are expanded. The most sensitive immunoassays for proteins detect the actual binding of the specific antibody with the epitope on the protein and do not rely on any secondary effects of that combination (such as complement activation or precipitation, for example). Techniques which measure this direct binding fall into one of two categories namely radioimmunoassay (RIA) and enzyme immunoassay (EIA). Both of these titles are generic terms which cover a whole range of different techniques. In RIA, the binding of antibody to the specific epitope is detected by a radiolabel which, depending on the technique, may be attached to the antigen or the antibody. Enzyme immunoassays utilize an enzyme which can convert a colourless substrate into a soluble coloured product which is measured spectrophotometrically. Usually, but not exclusively, the enzyme is attached to an antibody rather than to an antigen. Since the development of radio-immunoassay (RIA) antecedes enzyme immunoassays by several years, this will be discussed first.

RADIOIMMUNOASSAY

The most usual form of RIA is a competitive assay which was developed in 1968. This assay requires the following reagents:

- Radiolabelled antigen
- Unlabelled antigen
- Specific antibody

Pure antigen is needed both for radiolabelling, usually with an isotope of iodine, and to provide standard, known concentrations with which the 'unknown' can be compared. The assay works on the principle that a given amount of antibody (AB) will combine with a fixed amount of radiolabelled antigen (AG*) to produce a fixed amount of radiolabelled complex:

$$AB + AG^* \rightarrow ABAG^*$$

If, however, a known amount of unlabelled antigen were to be introduced into this system, the two forms of antigen would compete for the limited number of antibody combining sites with the result that some radiolabelled antigen would be 'displaced' from the complex. Thus there would be less radioactivity in the complex and a corresponding increase of radioactivity in the supernatant due to the displaced AG*:

$$AB + AG + AG^* \rightarrow ABAG + ABAG^* + AG^*$$

The more unlabelled AG is included, the less radiolabelled complex and the more free AG*. Thus, as long as the complex could be physically separated from the free antigen, a standard curve could be set up in which the amount of radiolabelled complex could be ascertained in the presence of increasing amounts of unlabelled antigen. Such a curve would look like Fig. 3.11 and could be used to determine the unknown concentration of an antigen preparation. Competitive radioimmunoassays of this type are very sensitive indeed, and can detect antigen in concentrations between 10^{-9} and 10^{-12} g/ml of solution.

A second type of RIA is based on a different principle. In this assay, antigen is absorbed onto the surface of a solid phase, usually the plastic of microwell plates. Protein antigens such as lymphokines are easily coated onto the surface of such

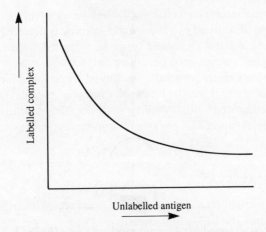

Fig. 3.11 Radioimmunoassay (RIA). Radioimmunoassay is a competitive inhibition assay based on the ability of unlabelled antigen to compete with labelled antigen for the binding sites on a limited number of antibody molecules. As the amount of unlabelled antigen is increased, the amount of radiolabelled complex decreases. The graph can then be used to determine the 'unknown' concentration.

plates by the use of a suitable 'coating buffer'. Following removal of any unbound antigen by washing, the bound antigen can be detected by the addition of specific antibody which is radiolabelled. Since the antibody is specific and will bind to antigen absorbed onto the solid phase, it follows that the more antigen bound, the more radioactivity will be bound also. This type of assay has almost limitless variations. For example, sensitivity may be increased if a two-stage procedure is used. In this case (see Fig. 3.12) the specific antibody (often a mouse monoclonal) is not radiolabelled. This unlabelled antibody can be detected by a second step in which, following appropriate washings, a radiolabelled anti-immunoglobulin is added. Alternatively, specific antibody may be bound first to the solid phase in order to 'capture' the antigen from a fluid in which it is present in such small quantities.

ENZYME IMMUNOASSAY

The most usual type of enzyme immunoassay is the enzyme-linked immunosorbent assay (ELISA) which most closely resembles the second type of RIA described above. Again, protein antigens are bound to a solid phase but the antibody used to detect it is labelled with an enzyme such as alkaline phosphatase or horseradish peroxidase. Again, the more antigen bound, the more antibody, and hence the more enzyme, will also be bound. A suitable chromogenic substrate is added and a colour reaction is allowed to develop for a limited period of time. The amount of product is measured spectrophotometrically and is

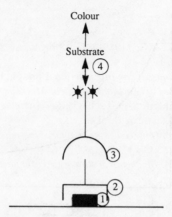

Fig. 3.12   Two-step enzyme-linked immunosorbent assay (ELISA). The plastic wells of a microtitre tray are coated with the protein to be estimated, (1) and incubated with an antibody to that protein. (2) After washing off excess antibody, the plate is incubated with an enzyme-labelled anti-immunoglobulin. (3) The enzyme is such that the addition of a substrate (4) produces a coloured product, the amount of which is measured by its ability to absorb visible light. The absorbance is then related to the amount of protein coating the wells.

directly related to the amount of antigen bound to the wells. ELISA techniques have been widely adopted since their inception in 1971 since they have none of the problems inherent in the use of radioactivity and the reagents have a longer shelf-life. However, it is probably fair to say that they are not as universally sensitive as competitive RIA and would most frequently be used to measure in the μg/ml to ng/ml range depending on the method.

Commercial immunoassay kits for lymphokines are now available from several well-known firms.

Summary

The biochemical characterization of lymphokines and interleukins has improved greatly in the last decade. In particular, gene cloning has allowed large amounts of recombinant protein to become available for analysis. In addition, rapid analytic and preparative separation procedures which have a high resolution have greatly improved the time in which a polypeptide can be sequenced by degradation of the protein or by prediction from the cDNA sequence. Knowledge of the number, distribution and affinity of lymphokine receptors has also increased although the mechanism of their action is still unproven. The receptors have binding affinities which, in most cases, approach those for hormone–receptor interactions.

References

Cole, C. R. and Smith, C. A. S. (1989). 'Glycoproteins: Structures and Functions', *Biochem. Educ.*, **17**, 179.

Edwards, R. (1985). *Immunoassay: an Introduction*. London, Heinemann Medical Books.

Lefkovitz, I. and Pernis, B. (1979). *Immunological Methods*. London, Academic Press.

Watson, J. D., Tooze, J. and Kurtz, D. T. (1983). *Recombinant DNA: A Short Course*. San Francisco, Scientific American Books.

Winnacker, E.-L. (1987). *From Genes to Clones: Introduction to Gene Technology*. Weinheim, New York, VCH.

Wrigglesworth, J. M. (1983). *Biochemical Research Techniques: A Practical Introduction*. Chichester, John Wiley.

4

Interleukin-1

Introduction

The name 'interleukin-1' (IL-1) describes two structurally related molecules, with similar activities *in vivo*. IL-1 promotes a variety of activities involved in inflammatory responses, including mediation of the 'acute phase response' – a rapid and non-specific response to infection and injury which is characterized by alterations in the levels of plasma proteins, blood phagocytes and body temperature. IL-1 is also involved in the initiation of specific immune mechanisms: it promotes activation of helper T-lymphocytes (T_H) following their interaction with antigen on the surface of antigen-presenting cells (APC) and also indirectly promotes the growth and differentiation of B-lymphocytes into plasma cells.

The discovery of IL-1 arose from studies on the conditioned media from cultures of adherent blood leukocytes. Peripheral blood mononuclear cells, obtained by fractionating blood on density gradients, can be readily separated into adherent and non-adherent fractions if the cells are incubated in plastic tissue culture flasks for about an hour. Monocytes form the bulk of the cells which adhere strongly to plastic whereas the lymphocytes are non-adherent. In 1972 the conditioned media from cultures of human peripheral blood adherent cells stimulated with lipopolysaccharide (LPS) for 24 h were found to contain a factor which promotes the proliferation of murine thymocytes (Gery *et al.*, 1972) treated with sub-optimal concentrations of lectins such as PHA (Fig. 4.1). The term 'lymphocyte activating factor' (LAF) was given to the, as yet, uncharacterized activity in these media. The discovery of LAF helped to provide some clue as to the role of monocytes and macrophages in the initiation of an immune response and in some circumstances LAF was able to substitute for these cells in eliciting immune responses *in vitro*. Since that time, a bewildering array of other

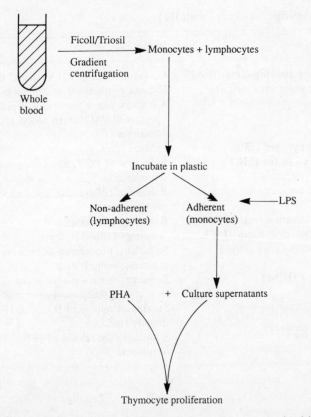

Fig. 4.1 Lymphocyte-activating factor (LAF). Monocytes are obtained by separation of whole blood on Ficoll/Triosil gradients, followed by incubation of the monocyte/lymphocyte preparation in plastic tissue culture flasks. The lymphocytes are non-adherent and can be separated from the adherent monocytes. When the monocytes are incubated with lipopolysaccharide, they release a factor into the medium which enhances the proliferation of thymocytes in the presence of PHA. This lymphocyte-activating factor was re-named interleukin-1 in 1979.

activities (Table 4.1) have been found to be associated with the same proteins (or their degradation products) that carry LAF activity. The recognition of the many different activities of LAF, on a range of target cells, led to the proposal, at the Second International Lymphokine Workshop, in 1979, that it be renamed 'Interleukin-1' (Aarden *et al.*, 1979). Several other interleukins have since been shown to have widespread effects on different cell types, a phenomenon known as 'pleiotropism', but few approach the range of activities demonstrated by IL-1.

Table 4.1   Activities associated with IL-1

Name of factor	Activity
Lymphocyte activating factor (LAF)	Co-stimulation of PHA-treated thymocytes
Leukocyte endogenous mediator (LEM)	Induces synthesis of acute phase proteins by hepatocytes; chemotaxis of polymorphs; egress of PMN from blood and bone marrow
Endogenous pyrogen (EP)	Induces fever
Monocytic cell factor (MCF)	Induction of PGE_2 and collagenase by synovial cells
Catabolin	Release of collagenase and destruction of cartilage matrix
Osteoclast activation factor (OAF)	Resorption of bone
Proteolysis inducing factor (PIF)	Wasting of muscles; fever
B-cell activation factor (BAF)	Stimulates production of immunoglobulin by antigen-specific B cells
Helper-peak 1 (HP-1)	Enhances *in vitro* plaque-forming cell response to sheep red blood cells
Tumoricidal activity	Stimulates release of IL-2 and IFN-γ; may be directly tumoricidal
Antiviral factor	Stimulates the release of IFN-β from fibroblasts

Biological activities of interleukin-1

Monocytes, macrophages and antigen-presenting cells generally are considered to be the major producers of IL-1 *in vivo* although many other cell types seem to have the capacity to produce it. Many microorganisms, including bacteria, yeasts and fungi, stimulate IL-1 production and endotoxins obtained from the cell walls of Gram-negative bacteria are particularly potent stimulators of its release. These endotoxins are lipopolysaccharides (LPS) (Fig. 4.2) and they induce IL-1 production at concentrations as low as 10^{-10} g/ml. Exotoxins produced by some Gram-positive bacteria can also elicit production of IL-1 and amongst these is the toxic shock syndrome toxin of *Staphylococcus aureus*. Moreover, antigen–antibody complexes and several activated complement components including C3b and C5a also stimulate IL-1 release. Macrophages have receptors for the Fc regions of complexed antibody as well as for C3b so that binding of macrophages to target cells is facilitated and phagocytosis and subsequent release of IL-1 promoted. C5a, which is produced in the lytic pathways, has a direct effect on macrophages, stimulating the release of IL-1. In this way, several

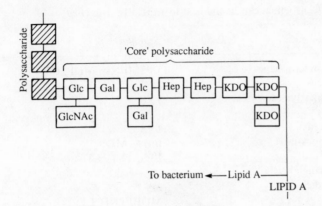

Fig. 4.2 The structure of lipopolysaccharide (LPS). The cell walls of Gram-negative bacteria contain considerable amounts of LPS which consists of repetitious polysaccharide linked to a 'core polysaccharide' which is in turn linked to a complex, saponifiable lipid component known as Lipid A. The core polysaccharide is shown below. In actual fact, the Lipid A component is the most active region in terms of stimulating inflammation. Key: Glc = glucose; GlcNAc = N-acetylglucose; Gal = galactose; Hep = heptose; KDO = 3-deoxy-D-manno-octulosonic acid. (See Westphal, 1975).

components generated by specific immune systems can promote acute phase inflammatory reactivity. In addition to the release of IL-1, phagocytosis of bacterial endotoxins can lead to the release of TNF-α by the same cells and these two molecules have many overlapping activities. A list of cells which can be induced to secrete IL-1 *in vitro* is given in Table 4.2.

Interleukin-1 is released from monocytes and macrophages following phago-cytosis of bacteria or bacterial products. Macrophages are concentrated in the tissues of the reticuloendothelial system (RES) and form part of the first line of defence against microorganisms. Extensive phagocytosis within this system results in the release of IL-1 into the blood and lymph. The levels of IL-1 in the plasma rise measurably even after localized inflammation and affect organs often at sites remote from the inflammation. Thus, IL-1 produced locally by cells in a lymph node draining an infected wound can exert a 'hormone-like' effect on cells in the liver, bone and brain. Recently, interest has centred on a membrane-bound form of IL-1 which is found at the surface of monocytes after they have been stimulated with LPS. It may well be that 'membrane' IL-1 and its soluble counterpart are responsible for different facets of its activities (Kurt-Jones *et al.*, 1978; Merluzzi *et al.*, 1987).

Table 4.2   Cells which can be induced to secrete IL-1 *in vitro*

Cellular sources	Stimulus*
Monocytes/macrophages	LPS, IFN-γ, MDP, C5a
Dendritic cells	LPS
Large granular lymphocytes	LPS
Astrocytes	LPS
Microglial cells	LPS
Skin keratinocytes	PMA, MDP
Endothelial cells	LPS, TNF, LT
Kidney mesangial cells	
Corneal epithelium	
Fibroblasts	MDP, TNF, LT
B-cell lines	Constitutive
Langerhans cells	LPS
P388D1 (murine macrophage line)	LPS, MDP
THP-1 (human monocyte line)	PHA, PMA, rTNF-α
U937.1 (human monocyte line)	LPS, MDP

* LPS = lipopolysaccharide; MDP = muramyl dipeptide; PHA = phytohaemagglutinin; TNF = tumour necrosis factor; PMA = phorbol myristate acetate.

IL-1 AND THE ACUTE PHASE RESPONSE

The acute phase response is a systemic reaction to infection which is characterized by alterations in the protein, amino acid and metallic ion content of the plasma (Table 4.3) and by fever. Shortly after the onset of an infection, hepatocytes in the liver are induced to switch from the production of serum albumin, to the synthesis of 'acute phase proteins', the concentration of which may be elevated several hundred-fold. Usually, the resolution of the infection marks the return to 'normal' levels. At least two other proteins are known to be involved in the production of an acute phase response and currently the relative contributions of IL-1, IL-6 and TNF-α are being evaluated (Fig. 4.3). Both recombinant IL-6 and IL-1 can induce similar responses when injected into experimental animals and it is known that the synthesis of IL-6 is induced by IL-1 *in vitro*. TNF-α is produced by macrophages under conditions similar to those which induce IL-1 production and recombinant TNF can induce some acute phase reactions *in vivo*. Moreover, both TNF-α and TNF-β (which is produced by antigen-stimulated helper T-lymphocytes) induce the synthesis of IL-1 by macrophages (Helle *et al.*, 1988; Ramadori *et al.*, 1988).

Acute phase reactants

The acute phase reaction is distinguished by dramatic changes in the levels of normal plasma proteins and by the production of proteins that are not usually detected in health. The role of some of these proteins remains obscure although

Table 4.3   Features of the acute phase response

Increase in plasma
Proteins
    C-reactive protein
    serum amyloid A
    fibrinogen
    haptoglobin
    α_1-antitrypsin
    caeruloplasmin
    some complement proteins
    α_1-macroglobulin
Amino acids – all types
Metallic ions – copper
Blood neutrophils

Decreases in plasma
Metallic ions – zinc, iron

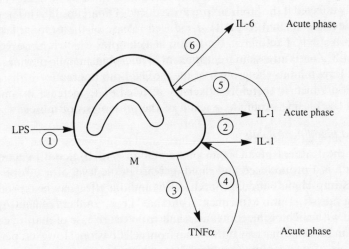

Fig. 4.3   Relationship between IL-1, IL-6 and TNF. Stimulation of macrophages
(M) with lipopolysaccharide (LPS) (1) results in the production of IL-1 (2). Tumour
necrosis factor (TNFα) is also produced (3) and this can in turn stimulate further
production of IL-1 (4). IL-1 also stimulates macrophages to produce IL-6 (5,6). All
three molecules induce acute phase responses in experimental animals.

others do have a clear role in the defence against infection. Levels of the C-reactive protein (CRP), for example, can rise several thousand-fold during infection, or experimental administration of IL-1. The binding of CRP to a pneumococcal protein can activate the complement via the classical pathway. Activation up to and including C3 stimulates phagocytosis of bacteria by PMNs and macrophages (Berman *et al.*, 1986). CRP is commonly found at inflammatory sites where it binds to the membranes and organelles of necrotic cells. Incomplete activation of the full lytic pathway beyond C3 may allow phagocytosis without further inflammation induced by activated C5. The concentration of serum amyloid A (SAA), a normal component of plasma, rises rapidly following administration of LPS to mice (Sipe *et al.*, 1979). The function of SAA in inflammation remains uncertain but constant elevation of this protein as a result of chronic inflammation may lead to the deposition of excess SAA or a cleavage product, amyloid A, in the tissues, resulting in a condition known as secondary amyloidosis. Fibrinogen is a normal plasma component with a well-documented role in the formation of a blood clot. Raised levels of fibrinogen can be detected within 5 h of administration of IL-1. The increased levels of the copper-binding protein, caeruloplasmin, are responsible for the increased plasma copper levels that are a standard feature of the acute phase response, and which are essential for the activity of several metalloenzymes involved in immune responses.

Other metabolic features which are characteristic of the acute phase response include lowered zinc and iron levels and an increase in blood amino acid levels. Iron is needed for all growing cells including microbes, the growth of which is adversely affected if the levels of iron are reduced (Dinarello, 1984). The decrease in iron levels is related to the IL-1-induced release of the protein, lactoferrin, from neutrophils. Lactoferrin binds iron in a complex which is removed by cells of the RES. Zinc is an essential component of microbial metalloenzymes so that a reduced level inhibits the growth of these cells. Both are required for microbial replication which is therefore adversely affected. The increase in amino acid levels in the plasma occurs as a result of the proteolysis of muscle.

IL-1 and blood neutrophils

One of the features of an acute phase response to bacterial infection or to endotoxin is a pronounced and rapid increase in the level of neutrophils in the blood (Kampschmidt and Upchurch, 1980) and this effect can be reproduced by injecting pure IL-1 into experimental animals. Peak numbers of neutrophils are achieved within 2 h of injection and result from the release of mature cells from reserves in the bone marrow rather than from cell division. However, persistently high levels of neutrophils (neutrophilia), which occurs as a result of chronic inflammation, are due to increased stimulation of the haemopoietic stem cells in the bone marrow. Several haemopoietic growth factors are released by T-lymphocytes during a specific immune response and the release of these is promoted indirectly by IL-1.

IL-1 and fever: the endogenous pyrogen

Fever is an alarming and consistent feature of bacterial and viral infection and can result in body temperatures up to 40°C. In young children, this may precipitate convulsions. Soluble factors have long been implicated in the induction of fever but for some years, the 'endogenous pyrogen' (EP) was thought to be a product of PMNs. Later, experiments of the type illustrated in Fig. 4.4 showed that the endogenous pyrogen is produced by monocytes and macrophages (Dinarello and Wolff, 1982). The endogenous pyrogen was found

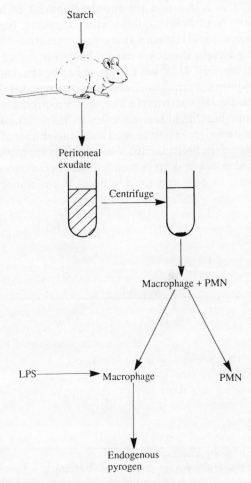

Fig. 4.4 Production of endogenous pyrogen. When mice are injected intraperitoneally with a starch solution, they produce a peritoneal exudate containing macrophages and polymorphonuclear leukocytes (PMNs). When these two populations of cells are separated, only the macrophages produce endogenous pyrogen when stimulated with lipopolysaccharide (LPS).

to be the same substance which is detected in the plasma of febrile rabbits and was identical to the LAF, and hence, IL-1.

It is now clear that many substances known to induce fever *in vivo*, do so by stimulating the release of IL-1 by mononuclear phagocytes. IL-1 induces fever through a direct effect on the temperature regulatory centre in the hypothalamus, possibly by stimulating the local production of prostaglandins, particularly PGE_2 (Fig. 4.5).

A clue to the immunological 'advantage' of fever probably lies in the fact that the high temperature present in a febrile patient favours the replication of lymphocytes and this is essential for the development of humoral and cell-mediated immunity. Neutrophil motility is also increased at higher temperatures, resulting in a more rapid inflammatory response. In addition, the higher temperatures may have a direct inhibitory effect on the growth of microbes themselves. Until recently, IL-1 was considered to be the major pyrogen in the host's immune response to infection, but it is now recognized that both TNF-α/β as well as IL-6 also have this activity. In fact, the fever-producing capacity of IL-1 may be entirely attributable to the induction of IL-6, although TNF can also induce fever in its own right (Helle *et al.*, 1988; Dinarello *et al.*, 1986). IL-1 also exerts other effects via the brain and these include the suppression of appetite and the induction of slow-wave sleep, which may conserve energy needed for the growth of the immune cells and the synthesis of antibodies and acute phase proteins.

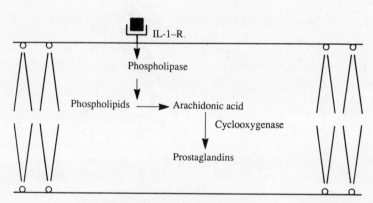

Fig. 4.5   IL-1 and prostaglandin production. IL-1 interacts with receptors (R) on the cell membrane resulting in the activation of phospholipase which cleaves the fatty acid moieties of membrane phospholipids. These fatty acids are rearranged to yield arachidonic acid which is converted into prostaglandins by the enzyme cyclooxygenase. Prostaglandins are probably responsible for the pyrogenic activity of IL-1.

Catabolic activities of IL-1

The injection of endotoxin into animals is followed by a sharp rise in the levels of amino acids in the blood (Baracos *et al.*, 1983). These amino acids are derived from IL-1-induced proteolysis of muscle and this can also be brought about by a 4 kDa degradation product of IL-1 known as proteolysis-inducing factor (PIF). The mechanism whereby IL-1 induces muscle proteolysis probably involves stimulation of the prostaglandin PGE_2 which activates the lysosomal proteases of neutrophils. In addition, the neutrophilia induced by IL-1 exacerbates this effect. Prolonged muscle breakdown in patients with chronic infections can lead to severe 'wasting' and this is probably a consequence of the combined activities of IL-1 and TNF (Dinarello *et al.*, 1986). In the short term, mobilization of amino acids from muscle may be beneficial for several reasons: patients with chronic infection have suppressed appetites so that increased oxidation of amino acids as a source of metabolic energy may be necessary. In addition, extra metabolic fuel is necessary to support the synthesis of the acute phase proteins by hepatocytes and to supply the energy requirements of proliferating haemopoietic and lymphoid cells. Other catabolic activities of IL-1 can be attributed to its induction of collagenase which can be demonstrated in cultured synovial cells (Krane *et al.*, 1982). IL-1 is present in the synovial fluids of patients with rheumatoid arthritis, a painful and debilitating autoimmune disease character-ized by chronic inflammation of the joints which are infiltrated with monocytes and lymphocytes, and by the presence of rheumatoid factor, an IgM antibody to IgG which is found in the blood and synovial fluids. Immune complexes of IgG and anti-IgG may be formed or deposited within the joints leading to local release of IL-1 and stimulation of collagenase by chondrocytes leading to destruction of the connective tissue in the joint. In addition, IL-1 has been identified as the osteoclast activation factor (OAF), originally discovered in the supernatants of activated lymphocytes, which stimulates the resorption of bone. Again, the consequences of bone resorption occurring over a period of time during long-term infections or in diseases such as rheumatoid arthritis where the acute phase response persists, can be crippling.

All of the features outlined above are host-generated and can be mimicked by injection, into healthy animals, of IL-1 or IL-1-containing sera from infected animals. While the acute phase response has a clear role in defence against microbial infection, it is also true that chronic stimulation of this response, which occurs in long-term infections such as tuberculosis, may result in tissue damage. In addition, chronic inflammatory disorders such as rheumatoid arthritis, where there is no proven microbial cause, are characterized by high levels of IL-1 and persistently high acute phase plasma protein levels.

It should now be obvious, from what has been discussed so far, that the effects of IL-1 in inducing an acute phase response are extremely ramifying. These effects, summarized in Fig. 4.6, are initiated as soon as a microorganism enters

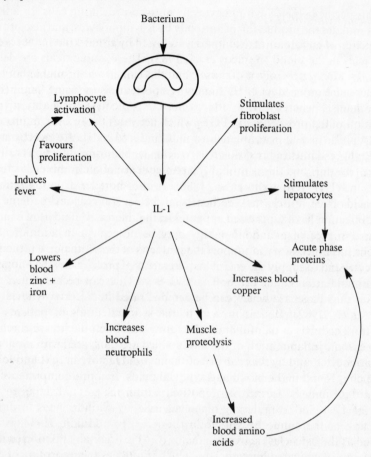

Fig. 4.6   IL-1 and the acute phase response. IL-1 has multiple activities on a range of cell types including fibroblasts, hepatocytes, muscle cells, bone marrow and brain cells. The proteolysis of muscle causes an increase in available amino acids, which are used by hepatocytes in the synthesis of acute phase proteins. High temperature favours lymphocyte proliferation and lowered blood iron and zinc levels inhibit replication of bacteria. The release of neutrophils from bone-marrow cells is responsible for the rapid rise in the number of these cells in the blood.

the body, and can be detected often within hours. What is not immediately detectable, but which is equally important, is the effect of IL-1 in the stimulation of specific immunity.

IL-1 and lymphocytes

The spectrum of activities promoted by IL-1 is not confined to the acute phase response since a major role of this interleukin is to promote the activation of antigen-specific helper T-lymphocytes by antigen-presenting cells. In addition, IL-1 stimulates the production of antibody by B-lymphocytes, and also promotes the activity of large granular lymphocytes having natural killer (NK) activity.

IL-1 and T-lymphocytes. IL-1 was first discovered as a soluble monocyte product which induced proliferation in thymocytes or lymphocytes treated with sub-optimal concentrations of PHA (Gery *et al.*, 1972). In addition, highly purified populations of lymphocytes are not stimulated, even with optimal doses of PHA, unless some macrophages or monocytes are added to the culture and IL-1 is able to substitute for macrophages under these conditions. IL-1 is also essential for antigen stimulation of lymphocytes although in this case it cannot replace APC. IL-1 stimulates the proliferation of antigen or lectin-stimulated lymphocytes by triggering the production, by helper T-lymphocytes, of the T-cell growth factor: IL-2 (Smith *et al.*, 1980). During the onset of a specific immune response, macrophages and other APCs process antigen which becomes inserted in the membrane in association with Class II molecules of major histocompatibility complex (MHC) (Fig. 4.7). This antigen–MHC complex is the first signal for the stimulation of the helper T-cell. IL-1 provides the second signal which results in the release, by the helper T-cell of IL-2. Whether IL-1 is essential for the release of IL-2, or simply enhances its release is a matter of some debate (Mizel, 1987; Oppenheim *et al.*, 1986). Macrophages which have been rendered incapable of producing IL-1 do not act as accessory cells *in vitro* unless exogenous IL-1 is added. Similarly, antibodies to IL-1 have been found to block the ability of normal macrophages to stimulate the proliferation of T_H in response to antigen. The release of IL-1 from macrophages may be triggered by membrane contact between the phagocytic cell and the microbe but internalization is needed for intracellular processing prior to re-exposure on the surface of the APC. T-cells themselves may be involved in a two-way stimulation process in

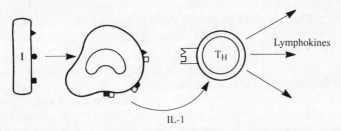

Fig. 4.7 Antigen presentation. IL-1 and activation of lymphocytes. An immunogen (I), depicted here with three different epitopes is taken up by an antigen-presenting cell and the epitopes expressed in the membrane in conjunction with Class II MHC antigen. The helper T cell (T_H) has specific receptors for this antigen/Class II complex and is stimulated to produce lymphokines providing that IL-1 is also produced by the antigen-presenting cells.

which interaction with antigen on the surface of APC causes the release of (uncharacterized) factors from T-cells, which stimulate release of IL-1 from macrophages. The two-way dependency of IL-1 release and T-cell activation could suggest interesting regulatory circuits having effects on both specific and non-specific immune mechanisms.

IL-1 and B-lymphocytes.   The term B-cell activation factor (BAF) was given to a soluble product of stimulated monocytes which could directly activate antibody-producing B-lymphocytes. When populations of spleen cells are depleted of T-lymphocytes, the remaining B-cells are unable to make an antibody response *in vitro*. However, BAF was found to restore to these lymphocytes the capacity to make specific antibody in the absence of T-cells (Wood and Cameron, 1976; Wood *et al.*, 1976; Falkoff *et al.*, 1984). Such results indicate that BAF (IL-1) can have a direct effect on B-lymphocytes. The helper T-cell is known to produce several factors which induce proliferation and differentiation of antigen-stimulated B-cells and IL-1 can synergize with these factors. Since IL-1 is effective during the early stages of activation its role may be to render the B-cell responsive to the growth and differentiation factors produced by T-cells. In support of this concept is the finding that highly purified B-lymphocytes which do not proliferate in response to the B-cell activator, pokeweed mitogen (PWM), can be triggered by a mixture of helper T-cell factors and IL-1. Antibody to IL-1 inhibits the generation of antibody-producing cells in response to polyclonal activators and the inhibitory effect can be reversed with pure IL-1 (Lipsky, 1985).

In addition to its role in B-cell activation, IL-1 may also be involved in the maturation of pre-B cells which can be distinguished from the mature B-cell by the absence of surface immunoglobulin. IL-1 has been shown to promote this maturation in pre-B-cell lines *in vitro*.

IL-1 and natural killer cells.   Natural killer (NK) cells are those cells which spontaneously lyse some tumour cell lines and virus-infected cells *in vitro*. NK activity is a property of blood leukocytes with the morphology of large granular lymphocytes (LGL) which comprise 5–10% of blood leukocytes. LGL-enriched fractions from human blood have been shown to be capable of producing abundant IL-1 (Scala *et al.*, 1984) and IL-1 synergizes with IL-2 in enhancing the tumoricidal affects of LGL (Ben-Aribia *et al.*, 1987) probably by inducing an increase in the expression of IL-2 receptors in these cells. The synergistic effects of IL-1 and IL-2 in increasing the cytotoxicity of NK cells may partially explain the antitumour activity of this protein although purified IL-1 is reported to have a direct tumoricidal action. In addition, when helper T-cells are stimulated by antigen and IL-1, they also release IFN-γ, which can stimulate the NK activity of LGL (Gidblund *et al.*, 1978; Henney *et al.*, 1981).

Interleukin-1 and disease

The inappropriate production of IL-1 has been implicated with IFN-γ in the development of autoimmune disease. Before a cell can present antigen to a helper

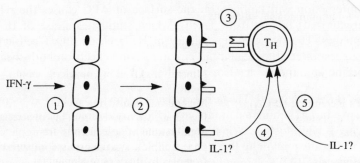

Fig. 4.8 IFN-γ and autoimmunity. A localized infection may result in local release of lymphokines (1), such as IFN-γ, which induce the expression of Class II MHC antigens on cells which do not normally express these (2). It is possible that these cells now present 'self' antigen to reactive helper T-cells (T_H) (3), which triggers an autoimmune reaction. IL-1 is also needed to stimulate these cells and possibly arises from macrophages at the site of the infection (5) although it cannot be ruled out that the 'induced' cells also release IL-1 (4).

T-lymphocyte, it must express Class II MHC antigens which are recognized by that T-cell. Class II antigens are confined to relatively few cells in the body compared with Class I antigens but many cells can be induced into expressing Class II by the lymphokine, IFN-γ. The induction of inappropriate Class II expression by IFN-γ could provide an explanation for several types of autoimmune disease, i.e. those diseases in which an individual produces an immune response against 'self' antigens (Bottazzo *et al.*, 1986). A local infection resulting in IFN-γ release from sensitized lymphocytes may induce expression of Class II determinants in bystander cells so that they effectively present 'self' antigen to specific helper T-cells, and trigger an autoimmune reaction (Fig. 4.8). The activated T_H in turn release more IFN-γ and amplify the problem. This theory presupposes that IL-1 is also available for stimulation of the helper T-cell. Abundant IL-1 can be found in the synovial fluid obtained from patients with rheumatoid arthritis and Class II expressing cells are also widespread (Klareskog *et al.*, 1982; Wood *et al.*, 1983). It is possible that immune complexes of rheumatoid factor combined with IgG may trigger IL-1 production by tissue macrophages rather than the synovial cells themselves. Other activities of IL-1 may have direct effects on tissue destruction, for example, by stimulation of prostaglandins and collagenase in the joints of patients with rheumatoid arthritis, or by induction of fibrotic areas in tissues which are the focus of chronic inflammation.

IL-1 plays an important role in wound healing because it stimulates the proliferation of fibroblasts from connective tissue. Fibroblasts are the first cells to emerge from a cut end of skin, for example, and their proliferation results in sealing of a wound. However, many diseases characterized by chronic inflammation result in fibrosis (scarring) of involved organs which is due to proliferation of fibroblasts attributable to IL-1 (Schmidt *et al.*, 1982).

Table 4.4   Immunological adjuvants

Adjuvant	Composition
Freund's complete (FCA)	Mineral oil, killed mycobacteria, emulsifying agent
Freund's incomplete (IFCA)	Mineral oil, emulsifying agent
Muramyl dipeptide	Peptidoglycan derived from mycobacteria
Liposomes	Membranous vesicles derived from phospholipids, antigen exposed on surface
Aluminium gels	Complex hydroxides of aluminium
Tuftsin	Tetrapeptide: Thre–Lys–Pro–Arg

Immunological adjuvants

An immunological adjuvant is a substance which, while not immunogenic *per se*, will increase the specific immune response when given with an immunogenic agent. They are extremely useful both experimentally and clinically for boosting responses to active immunization. A list of some common adjuvants is given in Table 4.4.

The mechanism of action of an adjuvant is not always the same and some may exert their effects by a combination of activities, the relative importance of each depending on the animal, the immunogen, and the method of administration. Some adjuvants may prolong the duration of an immune response by creating depots of immunogen which is released over a prolonged period of time. Many immunological adjuvants appear to boost non-specific immunity by promoting the synthesis and release of IL-1 by monocytes and macrophages. One of the most potent adjuvants is Freund's complete adjuvant (FCA) which is administered as a thick emulsion of the adjuvant and an aqueous solution of the immunogen. Mycobacteria which form part of FCA are potent stimulators of IL-1 and indeed the sites of injection with this adjuvant can become centres of intense inflammatory reactivity and granuloma formation which make FCA unsuitable for use in clinical immunization. Muramyl dipeptide (MDP) (N-acetyl muramyl-L-alanyl-D-isoglutamine), is the smallest structural unit of bacterial peptidoglycan which has adjuvant activity. Treatment of mouse macrophages *in vitro* with MDP results in IL-1 activity in cell supernatants, whereas analogues of MDP with no adjuvant activity *in vivo* fail to induce IL-1 *in vitro*.

Biochemistry of IL-1 and its receptor

PRODUCTION AND ASSAY

IL-1 can be detected in cultures of human monocytes within 60 min of stimulation with LPS. This production is inhibited by actinomycin D and cycloheximide, indicating *de novo* synthesis rather than pre-formed messenger. The ease with which monocytes can be stimulated by bacterial endotoxin, coupled with the ubiquity of endotoxin, can create experimental problems. For example, endotoxin is sometimes found in the sera used to supplement tissue culture media. Even sterilized plastic-ware may be contaminated since endotoxin is resistant to temperatures of 100°C and is active at very low concentrations. In order to study the effect of exogenous IL-1 in model systems it may be necessary to use polymyxin B, a cationic antibiotic which binds to the negatively charged LPS and inhibits its biological activities. Thus any effects seen in the system used can be attributed solely to the IL-1.

Recombinant IL-1, produced by cloning the gene in bacteria, is now widely available. Lack of glycosylation is not a problem because 'native' eukaryotic IL-1 does not appear to be modified in this way.

Regulation of IL-1 production

IL-1 increases the synthesis of the prostaglandin PGE_2 by activating membrane phospholipase enzymes. PGE_2 suppresses further production of IL-1 and this can be demonstrated by the addition of exogenous IL-1. The effect of PGE_2 is mediated via cyclic AMP, high levels inhibiting IL-1 release (Larrick, 1989). The release of IL-1 is also regulated by the phosphoinisitol (PIP) pathway since inhibition of protein kinase C also inhibits release of IL-1. Another feedback circuit for regulating IL-1 production concerns the interaction between IL-1 and the neuroendocrine system. IL-1 stimulates the production of several pituitary hormones including adrenocorticotrophic hormone (ACTH). ACTH stimulates the production by the adrenal glands of corticosteroids which inhibit IL-1 production. The anti-inflammatory properties of corticosteroids are well documented although the mechanism of action has remained uncertain until recently. Corticosteroids prevent the accumulation of neutrophils at inflammatory sites and also control fever and these effects may be explained by the inhibition of IL-1 production. In addition to the regulatory circuits already described, some naturally occurring inhibitors of IL-1 activity has been described. The urine of patients with monocytic leukaemia was found to contain a low molecular weight protein inhibitor of IL-1-induced PGE_2 production and which is most likely to be the product of the malignant monocytes. Normal macrophages are also reported to release IL-1 inhibitors after stimulation with immune complexes or some viruses. In particular, HIV-infected monocytes secrete large quantities of two distinct inhibitors which may contribute to the pathogenesis of this virus. The discovery of naturally occurring inhibitors of IL-1, and future discoveries concerning their mechanism of action, holds out hope for the treatment of chronic inflammatory disorders where the continued production of IL-1 contributes to the pathology of the disease.

Assay

The standard assay for IL-1 until recently was a bioassay based on the ability of IL-1 to stimulate thymocyte proliferation in the presence of sub-optimal concentrations of PHA. Since IL-1 is not species-specific, murine thymocytes (8–10 weeks) are frequently used. The assay has the advantage of being very sensitive but does not discriminate between other lymphokines such as IL-2 and IL-4 which have similar activities. IL-1 may be distinguished from IL-2 by its inability to support the growth of IL-2-dependent T-cell lines.

IL-1 is also sometimes measured by its ability to induce fever in rabbits and intravenous injection of IL-1 into rabbits will induce an increase in rectal temperature within 15 min. This assay is not recommended for IL-1 because it lacks sensitivity and requires far more IL-1 than is needed to support the proliferation of murine thymocytes. In addition, TNF and IL-6 also possess pyrogen activity. Other bioassays for IL-1 involve measuring plasma levels of iron, zinc, fibrinogen, or neutrophils following injection into rats. Similarly the production of acute-phase proteins by cultured hepatocytes will also provide an estimate of this activity. As yet, no bioassay will measure IL-1 exclusively so that immunoassays utilizing monoclonal antibodies to IL-1 are becoming much more widespread. Since IL-1 is not a single entity but a family of proteins, specific monoclonal antibodies to individual molecules allows the relative importance of each to be evaluated.

STRUCTURE OF IL-1

The evidence that all the activities attributed to IL-1 are, in fact, due to the same molecule comes from several sources. In particular, the fact that certain activities are inseparable despite extensive purification procedures is strongly indicative of a molecule with pleiotropic effects on inflammatory responses. For example, EP has been purified by gel filtration, affinity chromatography and ion-exchange chromatography and is always associated with LAF and leukocyte endogenous mediator (LEM) activity. Moreover, the spectrum of IL-1 activities shows identical sensitivity to chemical and physical agents and antibodies to LAF, for example, will remove EP activity from solution. IL-1 activity can be found in proteins with isoelectric points ranging from pI 4.0–8.0 and with molecular weights of 2–75 kDa. Nonetheless, two forms predominate and these are designated IL-1α and IL-1β. Complementary DNAs corresponding to proteins with IL-1 activity were first isolated in 1984 from human and mouse cells (Auron *et al.*, 1984; Lomedico *et al.*, 1984). Each correspond to a peptide of 31 kDa equivalent to a peptide of 269 and 270 amino acid residues, and with isoelectric pI values of 5.0 and 7.0, for the human and murine forms, respectively. Shortly after, cDNA corresponding to the murine IL-1 was isolated from human cells (March *et al.*, 1985). The properties of the two forms, IL-1α and IL-1β, are shown in Table 4.5.

The predominant extracellular form in each case is a 17 kDa peptide containing 150 amino acid residues. This 17 kDa protein represents the C-terminal 'half' of a 31 kDa precursor molecule which can be found in the cytoplasm of induced cells. An intermediate form, of 23 kDa, can be recovered

Table 4.5 A comparison of the biochemical and biological properties of IL-1α and IL-1β

Property	α	β
pI	5.0	7.0
Activity of 31 kDa precursor	Yes	No
Amino acids in precursor	270	269
Extracellular form	17 kDa	17 kDa
Predominant form in	Membrane	Blood and tissue fluids
Location of human gene	Unknown	Chromosome 2

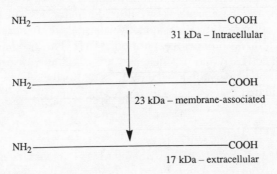

NH$_2$——————————————COOH
31 kDa – Intracellular

NH$_2$——————————————COOH
23 kDa – membrane-associated

NH$_2$——————————————COOH
17 kDa – extracellular

Fig. 4.9 Post-translational modification of IL-1. Newly synthesized IL-1 is a 31 kDa molecule which is cleaved at the membrane, where it appears as a 23 kDa form. This membrane-bound IL-1 may stimulate some activities of IL-1 which require cellular contact. An extracellular, 17 kDa, form has 'hormone-like activity'.

from stimulated cells by treatment with proteases such as trypsin (Fig. 4.9). Smaller extracellular forms probably represent degradation products of the 17 kDa molecule, whereas aggregates give rise to the larger molecular weight forms. One difference between the two forms is that the precursor of the α-form is biologically active whereas the precursor of the β-form is inactive and this absence of biological activity in the pre-processed IL-1β form correlates with its inability to bind to IL-1 receptors on the surface of sensitive cells. Human α- and β-forms show 26% homology for amino acid residues whereas the human and murine β-forms are almost identical.

One intriguing feature of IL-1 is the absence of a signal peptide on the newly synthesized protein. Most newly synthesized secretory proteins have a peptide of variable length at the N-terminal region of the molecule which eases passage across the endoplasmic reticulum and into the lumen (Fig. 4.10), prior to packaging of the molecule in the Golgi apparatus. The signal peptide has, typically, a charged end group which enables attachment to hydrophilic

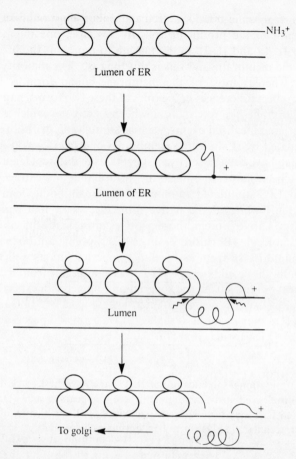

Fig. 4.10 Packaging of secretory protein into endoplasmic reticulum. Most secreted proteins are produced with a 'signal peptide' with a charged amino acid residue followed by a hydrophobic region. The charged residue interacts with the hydrophilic regions of the phospholipids in the endoplasmic reticulum (ER) membrane. As the peptide is synthesized, the hydrophobic signal sequence inserts through the ER and the signal peptide is cleaved within the lumen by proteases.

lipoproteins on the cytosol face of the endoplasmic reticulum, followed by a sequence rich in hydrophobic amino acids which are threaded through the lipid bilayer and into the lumen. Lacking a signal peptide, it is difficult to see how the protein is in fact secreted. Neither IL-1α or IL-1β are glycosylated and this tends to support the view that the molecule does not pass through the Golgi apparatus as is the usual case with secretory proteins. Moreover, the amino acid sequence of rIL-1 does not have an extensive hydrophobic region which would allow it to be inserted through the hydrophobic phospholipid bilayer. The mechanism whereby IL-1 leaves the cell is not at present known. It has been suggested that

IL-1 is really a membrane-bound molecule and that 'hormonal' IL-1 has been released on death of the producing cell. In this case, one might expect the proportions of IL-1α and IL-1β in the plasma to represent the proportions of each found in the membrane and this is not the case. The majority of secreted IL-1 is IL-1β whereas most of the membrane-bound form is IL-1α. This difference may reflect differences in the roles of these two forms, namely that IL-1β exerts the hormone-like role of IL-1 whereas activities which require close cellular contact, and localized events, such as stimulation of IL-2 release by T-cells, are stimulated by IL-1α in the membranes of APC (Conlon *et al.*, 1987).

Antisera which have been raised against peptides of different lengths obtained from IL-1 have been shown to bind to the intracellular and extracellular forms obtained from LPS-stimulated monocytes. Such antibodies can give some indication of the folding of the native molecule, since, if a peptide-specific antibody binds to native protein, those peptides must be presumed to be on the outside of the molecule (Bornford *et al.*, 1987). Specific antibodies have been used to precipitate IL-1β from extracellular supernatants as well as from cell lysates. The antibodies could precipitate a 35 kDa molecule from the cytoplasm, and two different peptides from the supernatant, namely, an expected 17.5 kDa molecule (mature IL-1β) as well as an intermediate form of 31 kDa. It has been suggested that IL-1 may be released as the 31 kDa form and processed externally to the active 17.5 kDa form.

MECHANISM OF ACTION

The IL-1 receptor

The biological effects of IL-1 are initiated when it binds to specific receptors on the surface of sensitive cells. The number of IL-1 binding sites on different cells is shown in Table 4.6. Figures obtained by following the binding of radiolabelled IL-1 to target cells do not always reflect the sensitivIty of that cell to the molecule. Indeed, some cells which are very sensitive to IL-1 do not even appear to bind measurable quantities of the radiolabel. T-lymphocytes have surprisingly few IL-1 receptors but it is possible that binding of IL-1 to a limited number of receptors may result in up-regulation of receptor expression as is known to occur

Table 4.6 Binding sites for IL-1

Cells	Binding sites
Fibroblasts	1500–5000
EBV transformed B-cells	200
Peripheral T-cells	50
LBRM 33/5A	500
EL4 thymoma	20 000

when IL-2 binds to specific receptor molecules on T-cells. In contrast, the murine EL4 thymoma cell line, which can secrete IL-2 after induction with IL-1, has 20 000 IL-1 receptors per cell (Lowenthal and Macdonald, 1986; Matsushima *et al.*, 1986). The large number of receptor sites on EL4 has made it an ideal cell for studying the binding affinities of the IL-1 receptor. The receptor molecules on EL4 cells are approximately 80 kDa in size and are heterogeneous with respect to binding affinities. Approximately 98–99% of receptors have a binding affinity (K_d) of $2–5 \times 10^{-10}$ M, i.e. this is the concentration of ligand which achieves 50% saturation of the receptors. The remaining 1–2% have affinities considerably higher – $K_d = 3–8 \times 10^{-12}$ M). A similar 'two-receptor' system is seen with IL-2.

The 80 kDa receptor of EL4 cells is a glycosylated molecule with a protein component which accounts for 65 kDa (Dower and Urdal, 1987). The latter has been cloned and analysed biochemically. It consists of a single polypeptide chain with >500 residues with a domain structure reminiscent of immunoglobulin. The external portion, consisting of >300 residues is anchored into the cell by a large cytoplasmic portion consisting of >200 residues, via a short hydrophobic transmembrane portion. Seven glycosylation sites are found in the extracellular portion of the molecule and these are thought to be important in the binding of IL-1, since minor changes in the carbohydrates can affect the binding affinity of the receptor. These differences might account for the two different affinities seen *in vitro* although a two-chain structure could also be proposed (Fig. 4.11). Currently, attempts are being made to uncover a second protein chain which might combine with the 80 kDa protein to form a high-affinity receptor (Dinarello *et al.*, 1989). IL-1α and IL1-β are known to use the same receptor although the binding affinities are sometimes different for the two forms. Unlabelled or 'cold' IL-1α can competitively inhibit the binding of radiolabelled IL-1β to target cells and vice versa. The utilization of the same receptors by pairs

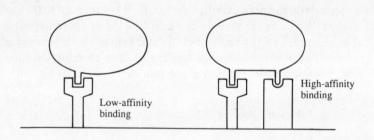

Fig. 4.11   Hypothetical two-chain structure of the IL-1 receptor. A single polypeptide chain can bind a ligand with low affinity. If the receptor is made up of two chains, each binding the ligand with a low or intermediate affinity, the result can be high-affinity binding. Thus, a single chain could be found in both the low- and the high-affinity receptor.

of structurally related molecules occurs amongst other cytokines, for example TNF-α and TNF-β, and IFN-α and IFN-β.

POST-BINDING EVENTS

IL-1, bound to cell surface receptors is internalized and has been found in the nucleus of treated fibroblasts (Bird and Sakhlatova, 1987). Whether or not this implies a direct effect of IL-1 on the regulation of target cells DNA is uncertain. It seems more likely that the effect of IL-1 is mediated by events stimulated at the membrane itself, so that a signal generated by ligand–receptor interaction is transduced across the membrane by enzymes such as phospholipases and protein kinases (Chapter 1). IL-1 has been shown to activate phospholipase A_2 in cultured rabbit chondrocytes (Chang *et al.*, 1986). Activation of phospholipases in cell membranes causes increases in membrane arachidonic acid which is available for conversion to prostaglandins via cyclooxygenase enzymes. Little is known about the effects of IL-1, on other systems for signal transmission across membranes, such as protein kinase C or the phosphoinositol pathway. The findings that some cells which are sensitive to very low concentrations of IL-1 do not bind measurable amounts of IL-1 and yet respond rapidly to it, is difficult to explain. If the IL-1 receptor consists of two polypeptide chains, it may be that binding to the 65 kDa chain on its own promotes internalization. On the other hand, binding to the second chain may be very low-affinity binding (and consequently not detected), and may initiate signal transduction as opposed to internalization.

Summary

Interleukin-1 is a fascinating molecule with multiple activities in immune responses. Through its effect on acute phase responses it promotes the synthesis of a range of proteins important in defence against microorganisms and affects plasma ion levels in ways which militate against bacterial replication. IL-1 is essential for the activation of T-lymphocytes and synergizes with other lymphokines in supporting the differentiation of specific antibody-producing cells. In addition, the fever which it induces via the hypothalamus favours lymphocyte proliferation, while muscle proteolysis stimulated by IL-1 provides the increased amino acid levels to support both lymphocyte division and the fibroblast activity necessary for wound healing. Much is known about IL-1-induced activities but its mechanism of action is as yet poorly understood. IL-1 is being increasingly implicated in pathological processes and its continued presence in long-term infections can result in chronic inflammation, leading to destruction of connective tissue, resorption of bone, muscle wasting, fibrosis and secondary amyloidosis. For these reasons, further study of the events which follow the binding of IL-1 to cell surface receptors are essential, since such knowledge could provide a rationale for treatment of these inflammatory disorders by blocking a crucial stage in these events.

References

Aarden, L. A., Brunner, T. K., Cerotinni, J-C. *et al.* (1979). 'Revised nomenclature for antigen non-specific T cell proliferation and helper factors', *J. Immunol.* **123**, p. 2928.

Auron, P. E., Webb, A. C., Rosenwasser, L. J. *et al.* (1984). 'Nucleotide sequence of human monocyte IL-1 precursor cDNA', *Proc. Natl Acad. Sci. (USA)* **81**, 7907.

Baracos, V., Rodemann, H. P., Dinarello, C. A. and Goldberg, A. L. (1983). 'Stimulation of muscle protein degradation and prostaglandin E_2 release by leukocytic pyrogen (interleukin 1). A mechanism for the increased degradation of muscle proteins during fever', *N. Engl. J. Med.* **308**, p. 553.

Ben-Aribia, M. H., Le Roy, E., Lantz, O. *et al.* (1987). 'Recombinant IL-2-induced proliferation of human circulating NK cells and T lymphocytes: synergistic effects of IL-1 and IL-2', *J. Immunol.* **139**, p. 443.

Berman, S., Gewurz, H. and Mold, C. (1986). 'Binding of C-reactive protein to nucleated cells leads to complement activation without cytolysis', *J. Immunol.* **136**, p. 1354.

Bird, T. A. and Sakhlatova, J. (1987). 'Studies on the fate of receptor-bound ^{125}I-IL-1β on porcine synovial fibroblasts', *J. Immunol.* **137**, p. 92.

Bornford, R., Abdulla, E., Hughes-Jenkins, C. *et al.* (1987). 'Antibodies to IL-1 raised with synthetic peptides: identification of external site and analysis of IL-1 synthesis in stimulated human peripheral blood monocytes', *Immunology* **62**, p. 543.

Bottazzo, G. F., Pujol-Barrell, R., Hanafusa, T. and Feldmann, M. (1986). 'Organ-specific autoimmunity: a 1986 overview', *Immunol. Rev.* **94**, p. 137.

Chang, J., Gilman, S. C. and Lewis, A. J. (1986). 'IL-1 activates phospholipase A_2 in rabbit chondrocytes: a possible signal for IL-1 action', *J. Immunol.* **136**, p. 1283.

Conlon, P. J., Grabstein, K. H., Alpert, A. *et al.* (1987). 'Localisation of human mononuclear cell IL-1', *J. Immunol.* **139**, p. 98.

Dinarello, C. A. (1984). 'Interleukin 1', *Rev. Infect. Dis.* **6**, p. 51.

Dinarello, C. A. and Wolff, S. M. (1982). 'Molecular basis of fever in humans', *Am. J. Med.* **72**, p. 799.

Dinarello, C. A., Cannon, J. G., Wolff, S. M. *et al.* (1986). 'Tumour necrosis factor (cachectin) is an endogenous pyrogen and induces production of IL-1', *J. Exp. Med.* **163**, p. 1433.

Dinarello, C. A., Clark, B. D., Puren, A. J. *et al.* (1989). 'The interleukin-1 receptor', *Immunol. Today* **10**, p. 49.

Dower, S. K. and Urdal, D. L. (1987). 'The interleukin-1 receptor', *Immunol. Today* **8**, p. 46.

Falkoff, R. J. M., Butler, J. L., Dinarello, C. A. and Fauci, A. S. (1984). 'Direct effects of a monoclonal B cell differentiation factor and of purified IL-1 on B cell differentiation', *J. Immunol.* **133**, p. 692.

Gery, I., Gershon, R. K. and Worksmen, B. H. (1972). 'Potentiation of the T lymphocyte response to mitogens: 1. The responding cell', *J. Exp. Med.* **136**, p. 128.

Gidblund, M., Orn, A., Wigzell, H. *et al.* (1978). 'Enhanced NK cell activity in mice injected with interferon and interferon-inducers', *Nature* **273**, p. 759.

Helle, M., Brakenhoff, J. P. J., De Groot, E. R. and Aarden, L. A. (1988). 'IL-6 is involved in IL-1-induced activities', *Eur. J. Immunol.* **18**, p. 957.

Henney, C. S., Kuribayashi, K., Kern, D. E., Gillis, S. (1981). 'Interleukin 2 augments natural killer cell activity', *Nature (London)* **291**, p. 335.

Kampschmidt, R. F. and Upchurch, H. F. (1980). 'Neutrophil release after injections of endotoxin or leukocyte endogenous mediator into rats', *J. Reticuloendothel. Soc.* **28**, p. 191.

Klareskog, L., Forsum, U. Scheynius, A. *et al.* (1982). 'Evidence in support of a self-perpetuating HLA-DR-dependent delayed-type cell reaction in rheumatoid arthritis', *Proc. Natl Acad. Sci. (USA)* **79**, p. 3632.

Krane, S. M., Goldring, S. R. and Dayer, J-M. (1982). 'Interactions among lymphocytes, monocytes, and other synovial cells in the rheumatoid synovium' in *Lymphokines*, Vol. 7, Eds Pick, E. and Landy, M., p. 75. New York, Academic Press.

Kurt-Jones, E. A., Fiers, W. and Pober, J. S. (1987). 'Membrane IL-1 induction on human endothelial cells and dermal fibroblasts', *J. Immunol.* **139**, p. 2317.

Larrick, J. W. (1989). 'Native interleukin 1 inhibitors', *Immunol. Today* **10**, p. 61.

Lipsky, P. E. (1985). 'Role of interleukin-1 in B cell activation', in *Contemporary Topics in Molecular Immunology* **10**, p. 195. London, Plenum Press.

Lomedico, P. T., Gubler, U., Hellman, C. P. *et al.* (1984). 'Cloning and expression of murine IL-1 cDNA in *Escherichia coli*', *Nature (London)* **312**, p. 458.

Lowenthal, J. W. and Macdonald, H. R. (1986). 'Binding and internalisation of IL-1 by T cells. Direct evidence for high and low affinity classes of IL-1 receptor', *J. Exp. Med.* **164**, p. 1060.

March, C., Mosley, B., Alf, L. *et al.* (1985). 'Cloning, sequence and expression of two distinct human IL-1 cDNAs', *Nature (London)* **315**, p. 641.

Matsushima, K., Akatioshi, T., Yamada, M. *et al.* (1986). 'Properties of a specific IL-1 receptor on human Epstein–Barr virus-transformed B lymphocytes: identity of the receptor for IL-1α and IL-1β, *J. Immunol.* **136**, p. 4496.

Merluzzi, V. J., Faanes, R. B., Czajkowsky, M. *et al.* (1987). 'Membrane-associated IL-1 activity on human U937 tumour cells: stimulation of PGE$_2$ production by human chondrosarcoma cells', *J. Immunol.* **139**, p. 166.

Mizel, S. B. (1987). 'Interleukin 1 and T cell activation', *Immunol. Today* **8**, p. 330.

Oppenheim, J. J., Kovacs, E. J., Matsushima, K. and Durum, S. K. (1986). 'There is more than one interleukin 1', *Immunol. Today* **7**, p. 45.

Ramadori, G., Van Damme, J., Rieder, H. and Meyer zum Buschenfelde, K.-H. (1988). 'IL-6, the third mediator of the acute phase reaction, modulates hepatic protein synthesis in humans and the mouse. Comparison with IL-1β and TNFα', *Eur. J. Immunol.* **18**, p. 1259.

Scala, G., Allavena, P. Djeu, J. Y. *et al.* (1984). 'Human LGLs are potent producers of IL-1', *Nature (London)* **309**, p. 56.

Schmidt, J. A., Mizel, B. L., Cohen, D. and Green, I. (1982). 'Interleukin 1, a potent regulator of fibroblast proliferation', *J. Immunol.* **128**, p. 2177.

Sipe, J. D., Vogel, S. N., Ryan, J. L., McAdam, K. P. W. J. and Rosenstreich, D. L. (1979). 'Detection of a mediator derived from endotoxin-stimulated macrophages that induces the acute phase serum amyloid A response in mice', *J. Exp. Med.* **150**, p. 597.

Smith, K. A., Gilbride, K. J. and Favata, M. F. (1980). 'Lymphocyte activating factor promotes T cell growth factor production by cloned murine lymphoma cells', *Nature (London)* **287**, p. 353.

Westphal, O. (1975). 'Bacterial Endotoxins, the second Carl Prausnitz Memorial Lecture', *Int. Arch. Allergy. Appl. Immunol.* **49**, pp. 1–43.

Wood, D. D. and Cameron, P. M. (1976). 'Stimulation of the release of a B-cell activating factor from human monocytes', *Cell. Immunol.* **21**, p. 133.

Wood, D. D., Cameron, P. M., Poe, M. T. and Morriss, C. A. (1976). 'Resolution of a factor that enhances the antibody response of T cell depleted murine splenocytes from several other monocyte products cell', *Immunology* **121**, p. 188.

Wood, D. D., Ihrie, E. J., Dinarello, A. A. and Cohen, P. L. (1983). 'Isolation of an interleukin 1-like factor from human joint effusions', *Arthritis Rheum.* **26**, p. 975.

5

Interleukin-2

Introduction

The 1970s witnessed an explosion of interest in the production of long-term cultures of lymphocytes. The benefits of cultures of stimulated B-cells, producing unlimited quantities of monoclonal antibodies of pre-defined specificity were realized in 1975 (Kohler and Milstein, 1975), although it was found necessary to 'immortalize' the activated B-cells by hybridization with cultured myeloma cells. Such monoclonal antibodies have revolutionized the study of biology in general and immunology in particular and have found many industrial and clinical applications. Less predictable, perhaps, were the benefits of long-term cultures of stimulated T-cells but amongst other things, such cultures might allow the clonal analysis of the cells of the immune response and of their products. The protein products of activated T-lymphocytes might then be used as a source of lymphokines with clinical potential, for example, in replacement therapy for patients suffering from immunodeficiency disease.

T-cells can readily be stimulated *in vitro* by one of several methods. These methods have already been described in Chapter 2 so that a very brief outline should suffice.

(1) Several plant lectins are mitogenic for lymphocytes and, in particular, phytohaemagglutinin (PHA) and concanavalin A (Con-A) stimulate the proliferation of T-cells. The stimulation is polyclonal but stimulated cells could, in theory, be cloned following lectin treatment. Stimulation of T-cells with lectins requires the presence of accessory cells (macrophages) or the IL-1 which they produce. The stimulation is rapid: there is a peak of cell division after 3 days as measured by the incorporation of tritiated thymidine into DNA. Unfortunately, such cultures inevitably fail after 10–12 days and the new cells die.

(2) Allogeneic populations of lymphocytes will stimulate each other to proliferate in the mixed lymphocyte reaction (MLR) and if one of the populations is irradiated, only the second population will proliferate. The growth of T-cells in an MLR is again disappointingly short-lived and the cells rapidly die out.

(3) Immune lymphocytes can be stimulated *in vitro* by culture with the appropriate antigen. For example, lymphocytes obtained from someone immune to *Mycobacterium tuberculosis* would proliferate *in vitro* in response to the bacterium or to a purified protein derivative (PPD) of the organism. Macrophages are essential for presentation of antigen and only the antigen-specific cells will respond.

Most early attempts at long-term culture of T-lymphocytes used PHA to activate the lymphocytes since prior immunization was not necessary. A major breakthrough came in 1976, when it was discovered that T-cells could be maintained indefinitely in culture if the growth medium was supplemented at regular intervals with fresh supernatants from PHA-stimulated cultures (Fig. 5.1). The growth-promoting activity of these 'conditioned media' was not due to residual PHA which could be removed by affinity chromatography, and was instead attributed to a putative T-cell growth factor (TCGF) (Morgan *et al.*, 1976). The discovery of TCGF led to the production of T-cell clones using either PHA or specific antigen to stimulate the cells, and the techniques of limiting

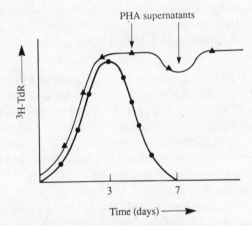

Fig. 5.1 PHA stimulation of T-lymphocytes. PHA is a non-specific stimulator of T-lymphocytes and induces a rapid proliferation in these cells. The growth of stimulated cells can be measured by the uptake of tritiated thymidine (^{3}H-TdR) into the DNA. PHA-stimulated lymphocytes rapidly die out after the initial proliferation due to depletion of the available T-cell growth factor, TCGF (●), but can be induced to proliferate further if regularly supplied with the supernatants from freshly stimulated cultures (▲) which contain TCGF.

dilution. These developments were aided by parallel developments in mono-clonal antibody technology whereby antibodies became available which could discriminate between the T-cell subsets, enabling initial cell populations to be separated to a high degree of purity with the fluorescence-activated cell sorter (FACS) and also allowing the clonal products to be phenotyped.

In 1979, TCGF was re-named as interleukin-2 (IL-2) in response to an increasing awareness of its central role in the production of an effective immune response (Aarden *et al.*, 1979). For example, it was found that animals which were injected with antibodies to IL-2 suffered a profound immunosuppression. Similarly, the highly potent immunosuppressive fungal peptide, cyclosporin A, which was being used to prevent the rejection of transplants in humans, was shown to inhibit the synthesis of IL-2 by activated T-lymphocytes *in vitro*. IL-2 was subsequently shown to be essential for the development of both cell-mediated and humoral immunity and well as stimulating the killing of tumours by NK cells. The activity of IL-2 in promoting tumour cell killing has led to extensive clinical trials, and the recognition that treatments utilizing this protein, though not without problems of toxicity, have indeed led to clinical remission of tumours.

Role of IL-2

IL-2 is produced principally by T-cells belonging to the helper/inducer subset, the stimulus for production being the recognition of antigen on the surface of antigen-presenting cells (APC) as a complex with Class II molecules of the MHC. Natural killer cells also produce IL-2 *in vitro* in response to exogenous IL-2 or to IL-2 generated *in situ* by activated T-cells. The role of IL-2 can be summarized as follows:

(1)   As a growth factor, it supports the proliferation and differentiation of any cells which have high affinity IL-2 receptors for it. Resting (unstimulated) T-lymphocytes belonging to either the helper or cytotoxic subsets possess few of these receptors, but following stimulation with specific antigen or with mitogen, the number increases substantially. Combination of IL-2 with its specific receptor on antigen-stimulated T-cells induces proliferation and functional differentiation in those cells. Thus, IL-2 is essential for the full development of cytotoxic T-lymphocytes which are important in antiviral immune responses. In addition, binding of IL-2 to receptors on T_H stimulates not only the proliferation of these cells but also the sequential release of other lymphokines. The specificity of the response is maintained by the interaction of antigen with specific antigen receptors on the surface of the responding T-cells (Fig. 5.2).

(2)   More recently (Meidema and Melief, 1985) it has been shown that B-lymphocytes also respond to antigen by producing IL-2 receptors. Similarly, they can be induced to express the appropriate receptors

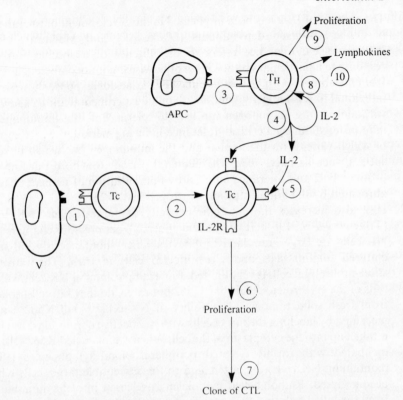

Fig. 5.2 Role of IL-2 in the development of cytotoxic T-lymphocytes (CTL). (1) A CD8$^+$ cell, Tc, recognizes specific viral antigen on the surface of an infected cell in associated with Class I MHC determinants. (2) The Tc starts to produce, and express, cell surface receptors for IL-2. (3) Presentation of antigen by an APC to a specific helper T-cell (T$_H$) which (4) initiates the release of IL-2 by these cells. (5) IL-2 binds to the receptors on antigen-stimulated Tc causing them to (6) proliferate and differentiate to produce a clone of CTL (7). (8) IL-2 can also auto-stimulate the T$_H$ to (9) proliferate and (10) to release other lymphokines.

following stimulation with lectins such as pokeweed mitogen (PWM) which stimulate B-cells. PWM-induced proliferation of B-cells requires the presence of IL-2 supplied by helper T-cells. However, other factors, such as IL-4, are also required for the full differentiation of B-cells into antibody-secreting plasma cells and there is evidence that the release of such factors from helper cells is promoted by IL-2 (Robb, 1984). Experimental evidence obtained by the cloning of helper T-cells in mice has suggested that IL-2 and interleukins 4 and 5 are produced by different helper T-cells and influence the production of different classes and subclasses of antibodies (Mosmann and Coffman, 1987). In humans there is little evidence so far that these are mutually exclusive products.

(3)   The absence of IL-2 has been implicated in the development of tolerance to particular antigenic determinants (Malkowsky and Medawar, 1984). Immunological tolerance refers to the absence of a specific antibody response to a particular epitope in an otherwise immunocompetent animal. It is a phenomenon which is exemplified by the lack of response shown by an individual to self-antigens. Immunization of experimental animals *in utero* with almost any immunogen can lead to tolerance if that immunogen is administered during a critical 'tolerance-inducing' period, the precise span of which varies with the animal and the immunogen but which in some species, such as mice, spans the neonatal period. Newborn mice do not produce IL-2 and tolerance induced by immunization of neonates can be abrogated by the administration of exogenous IL-2.

(4)   IL-2 also increases the cytotoxic capacity of natural killer (NK) cells (Trinchieri *et al.*, 1984). It will be remembered from previous chapters that NK cells are large granular lymphocytes which spontaneously kill some cultured tumour cells and virus-infected cells *in vitro*. The range of susceptible target cells is very limited. For example, human NK cells will kill cells of the erythroleukaemic line K562 but rarely do they kill cells isolated from fresh solid tumours. The ability of NK cells to kill K562 can be measured by labelling the target cells with radioactive chromium-51, which is taken up into the cytoplasm of the cell. When radiolabelled K562 cells are incubated with freshly isolated peripheral blood lymphocytes (PBL) (containing NK cells) the latter bind to the susceptible target cells which become lysed. Radiolabelled cytoplasm is released into the supernatant from the killed cells and the amount of radiolabel indicates the number of cells killed. In practice, the released label is compared with the release from labelled cells incubated in the absence of NK cells and both are expressed as a proportion of the total counts which can be released from cells following treatment with a detergent such as Triton X100. Thus:

Percentage cytotoxicity =

$$\frac{[\text{Total counts (Triton)}] - [\text{Counts in test}]}{[\text{Total counts (Triton)}] - [\text{Spontaneous release}]} \times 100$$

If PBL are incubated for at least 1 h with IL-2, the cytotoxicity of the NK cells is dramatically increased (Fig. 5.3), although the range of susceptible targets remains the same. When NK cells are treated with IL-2 they start to produce IFN-γ which is also known to increase the cytotoxicity of these cells. However, the effect of IL-2 on NK activity cannot be entirely attributed to the synthesis of IFN-γ because the increase in cytotoxicity still occurs even in the presence of antibodies to IFN-γ. Instead, IL-2-mediated increases in cytotoxicity may be the result of IL-2 promoting the maturation of immature NK cells into the fully functional state, with a corresponding increase in cytotoxicity within a fixed population.

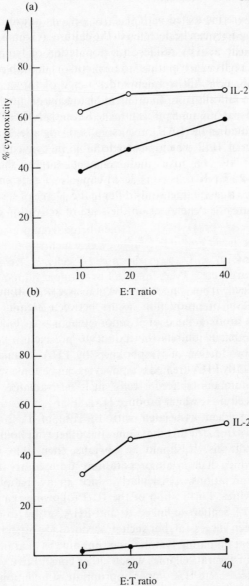

Fig. 5.3 IL-2 and natural killer cells. The two graphs show the cytotoxicity of peripheral blood NK cells for an NK-sensitive target cell, the erythroleukaemia, K562. Both graphs show the killing of ^{51}Cr-labelled target cells at effector:target ratios of 10, 20 and 40:1, respectively. In both cases, overnight preincubation of lymphocytes with IL-2 increases the cytotoxicity but this is more evident in lymphocytes obtained from individuals who have a naturally low level of NK activity (b). In (a) the difference is less marked simply because the resting level is quite high (possibly because of a recent infection).

(5) When PBL are incubated with IL-2 for periods in excess of 48 h, a fresh cytotoxic capacity can be detected in the cultures (Grimm *et al.*, 1982). This 'new' cytotoxic activity resides in a population of lymphokine-activated killer (LAK) cells which mature from precursors in the blood and lymphoid tissues. LAK cells kill a much wider range of target including freshly isolated tumour cells from a variety of histogenic origins, and fetal cells, as well as the usual NK susceptible targets. Recently NK cells have themselves been implicated as the LAK precursors, showing a level of cytotoxicity in the absence of IL-2 which is undetectable in conventional assays. The concept of NK 'sensitive' and 'resistant' targets should perhaps be abandoned and NK cells considered capable of different states of activation. In such a case, targets only differ in the degree of susceptibility to lysis and this in turn is dependent on the state of activation of the lytic cells.

Sources of IL-2

IL-2 can be produced from lymphocytes which have been stimulated with PHA. The maximum level of production occurs between 24 and 48 h and can be enhanced if cells are irradiated or if indomethacin is included in the culture medium. Indomethacin inhibits the monocyte production of prostaglandins which suppress production of lymphokines by PHA-stimulated T-cells. The production of IL-2 by PHA-treated lymphocytes can be considerably elevated by including small numbers of 'feeder cells' such as irradiated leukocytes or B-lymphoblastoid cell lines which produce IL-1.

The biggest problem associated with the use of IL-2 from stimulated lymphocytes arises from the fact that numerous other lymphokines are produced under these conditions. It should be obvious, then, that the results from experiments in which such crude preparations are used are always subject to alternative interpretations, particularly since many lymphokines mediate overlapping activities. Purification of the IL-2 following removal of PHA on affinity columns of Sepharose linked to anti-PHA, or by absorption onto red blood cells has been successful, but such procedures are often laborious and the removal of all contaminating lymphokines not always guaranteed. The fortuitous discoveries of several cell lines which either constitutively produce IL-2 or can be induced to secrete IL-2 under appropriate stimulation, meant that the lymphokine could be produced in larger quantities although not necessarily in a purer form. For example the gibbon lymphoblastoid cell line MLA 144 (Clark and Kamen, 1987), derived from a spontaneous lymphosarcoma, produces IL-2 constitutively but has more recently also been shown to secrete IL-3. The JURKAT line, derived from a human T-cell lymphoma, secretes IL-2 after stimulation with phorbol esters and/or lectins and production levels of 1000 U IL-2/ml of culture medium have been measured following stimulation with Con-A. However, IL-2, like many lymphokines is measured in 'units of activity' which are related to specific bioassays and, since all lymphokines have a very high specific activity, 1000 U/ml correspond to nanogram quantities of protein. Such tiny amounts are not easily purified from other, equally active, molecules which are also present in the same low concentrations.

In recent years, pure recombinant IL-2 has been produced by cloning the IL-2 gene from stimulated JURKAT cells and expressing them in mammalian cells or in bacteria (Taniguchi *et al.*, 1983). Recombinant human (rHu) IL-2 is now used clinically for cancer therapy and immune replacement therapy but many laboratories still use partially purified MLA 144 extracts for T-cell cloning, not the least because of its relative cheapness.

Assay of IL-2

The advent of the purer recombinant form has also allowed quantification of the activity of the molecule which is shown to be active at the ng/ml level. Nonetheless, IL-2 is more generally measured as 'units of activity' in one of the following bioassays:

(1) The ability to support the proliferation of lectin-stimulated cultures of PBL.
(2) The ability to support the proliferation of lectin-stimulated thymocytes. However, since this method also assays IL-1 and IL-4, it is probably best avoided.
(3) The ability to support the growth of IL-2-dependent cultured T-lymphocyte lines (CTLL). This system is relatively sensitive and several murine CTLL are available which respond to human IL-2.

Whenever IL-2 is used for the first time, and particularly if it has been purified from stimulated T-cells or T-cell lines, it is a good idea to titrate the IL-2 to establish optimal doses in the system used. Ideally, published units of activity should be compared to a standard reference sample or specific activities given, but this is not always the case.

Molecular biology

In humans, IL-2 is encoded by a single, non-allelic gene on the long arm of chromosome 4 (4q) (Robb *et al.*, 1984). The primary translation product is a polypeptide of 153 amino acids which includes a signal peptide of 20 amino acid residues. Figure 5.4 shows the molecule arbitrarily folded. Reduction of the single disulphide linkage between cysteine residues 58 and 105 with mercapto-ethanol results in complete loss of biological activity. Differences in the properties of human IL-2 secreted by different cells under varying conditions are entirely attributable to post-translational glycosylations. A single O-glycosylation site is found at residue 3 which is occupied by threonine. Differences in

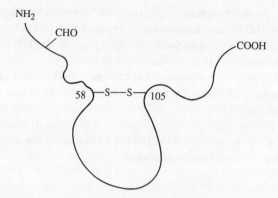

Fig. 5.4 Structure of IL-2. The IL-2 molecule is a single polypeptide chain of 133 amino acid residues. The molecule is O-glycosylated at residue 3 which is threonine, and an essential disulphide link is found between residues 58 and 105. A single gene exists for IL-2 so that differences in molecular species are entirely attributable to different degrees of glycosylation.

O-glycosylation at this site result in a range of molecular weights of 15–17 kDa for the mature molecule and p*I* values ranging from the frankly acid (pH 4.2) to mildly alkaline (pH 8.2). IL-2 produced by human PBL or tonsillar lymphocytes is a mixture of unglycosylated molecules and species with O-linked galactosamine, galactose and sialic acid whereas JURKAT IL-2 is either unglycosylated or has a single attached galactosamine residue. Recombinant IL-2, produced in *E. coli*, has all the activity of the lymphocyte-derived molecule despite lack of glycosylation. To date, no biological activity has been ascribed to the carbohydrate although a number of ideas have been proposed: it may, for example, be significant in prolonging the half-life in extracellular fluid or may affect its transport by altering the isoelectric points. Recent evidence, for example, using recombinant IL-3 has shown a profound effect of glycosylation on the distribution rate of the molecule in body fluids (see Chapter 6). Mouse IL-2 shows a 60% sequence homology with human IL-2 and this similarity is reflected in the ability of IL-2 to promote the growth of several mouse T-cell lines. Mouse IL-2 separated by SDS–PAGE has an apparent molecular weight of 32 kDa, indicating that it may exist as a dimer.

Attempts to identify fragments of IL-2 with biological activity, by selective enzymic degradation have not resulted in any active fragments but it is possible that the wider availability of the recombinant molecule and the development of new technologies in molecular biology, such as site-directed mutagenesis, will allow minor alterations in the primary structure of the protein to be investigated.

IL-2 RECEPTORS

Interleukin-2 exerts its biological effects by combination with cell surface receptors and in this respect it closely resembles other hormone/receptor systems.

The binding is characteristically of high affinity, shows saturation kinetics and is specific. Radiolabelled IL-2 will bind to the surface of PHA-activated blasts with a dissociation constant (K_d) of between 10^{-11} M and 10^{-12} M. Binding can be shown to occur within 48 h of stimulation with PHA coincident with the appearance of the receptors. The expression of IL-2 receptors reaches a maximum between 3 and 5 days following PHA stimulation (Fig. 5.5) but decline thereafter unless the cells are re-stimulated with fresh lectin (Cantrell and Smith, 1983).

Studies on the IL-2 receptor were greatly facilitated by the production in 1981 of a monoclonal antibody which appeared to bind to an epitope on the receptor itself (Uchiyama *et al.*, 1981). The antibody was produced by immunizing mice with cultured human T-cells from a patient with cutaneous T-cell lymphoma and was shown to bind to cell lines of similar derivation, and to lectin-stimulated T-cells but not to 'resting' T- or B-cells from peripheral blood. The monoclonal antibody was called Anti-Tac because it identified *act*ivated *T* cells and the glycoprotein to which it bound the 'Tac' protein. Anti-Tac was also shown to block the growth-promoting effects of IL-2, and to compete with radiolabelled IL-2 for binding sites on PHA blasts, indicating that it identified an epitope present on the IL-2 receptor.

The kinetics of binding of Anti-Tac and radiolabelled IL-2 to stimulated cells are essentially the same but some interesting differences have emerged in the estimates of the numbers of binding sites on cell surfaces. Whereas the binding of radiolabelled IL-2 to activated cells indicated between 2000 and 4000 sites per cell, the binding of Anti-Tac indicated a much higher number of receptors (30 000–60 000). One hypothesis which has gained much support suggests that

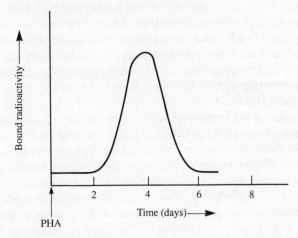

Fig. 5.5 Binding of radiolabelled IL-2 to PHA-stimulated lymphocytes. Resting lymphocytes express few high-affinity receptors for IL-2 but can be detected within 48 h of stimulation with PHA. The binding of radiolabelled IL-2 to stimulated cells reaches a peak at 3–5 days and then declines.

this figure represents the sum of high- and low-affinity receptors both of which contain the Tac epitope. The very low concentrations of radiolabelled IL-2 used in the binding assays, and which were chosen because they were known to produce growth stimulation, would only detect receptors of high affinity. In fact, when radiolabelled IL-2 is used at concentrations 1000 times·higher, then the number of binding sites is closer to that obtained by Anti-Tac binding. The Tac glycoprotein has been characterized following isolation from detergent-solubilized cells by affinity binding to immobilized Anti-Tac. It is a single polypeptide chain made up of 272 amino acids, including a signal sequence of 21 amino acids, a transmembrane hydrophobic region of 19 amino acids and a very short cytoplasmic sequence of 13 amino acids. It is the product of a single structural gene located on chromosome 10 in humans and the protein component has a molecular weight (after removal of a signal peptide) of 33 kDa. The protein is both N- and O-glycosylated, which gives it a molecular weight of 55 kDa, phosphorylated (at the serine residue at position 247), and sulphated. Resting T-cells do not have mRNA specifying the Tac protein but this can be detected within 3 h of activation with mitogen. Production of mRNA peaks at 24 h although expression of the protein itself does not peak until 48–72 h (Greene and Robb, 1985).

Recently, a 75 kDa IL-2 binding protein (p75) has been found which binds IL-2 with an intermediate affinity ($K_d = 10^{-9}$ M) (Smith, 1987). The protein was originally discovered on a cell line derived from a patient with T-cell acute lymphoblastic leukaemia (T-ALL). These cells also express the Tac protein but after cloning, some clones were found to have both low- and high affinity receptors, while others bound IL-2 with the intermediate affinity but failed to bind Anti-Tac. The sole IL-2 binding protein in these cells was p75. Analysis of all clones revealed that only those clones which expressed both proteins were able to bind IL-2 with high affinity. Since then, the p75 protein has been found on normal, stimulated T-cells, and the high-affinity receptor is considered to be a heterodimer of both of these proteins whereas the Tac antigen alone binds only with the low-affinity receptor (Fig. 5.6). The designation of p75 and p55 as α and β follow the convention of naming other cell surface receptors in which the larger polypeptide chain is named α.

The significance of the large number of Tac molecules on activated cells is not fully understood although it has been suggested that soluble Tac, released from activated cells, may regulate the amount of IL-2 in the circulation. Whereas binding to high-affinity receptors is absolutely necessary for the proliferative responses in T- and B-cells, it may be that binding to Tac proteins can stimulate the release of other lymphokines without inducing proliferation. NK cells, which develop increased cytotoxicity in the presence of IL-2, do not express the Tac molecule and Anti-Tac does not inhibit IL-2-induced proliferation and increased cytotoxicity. It is assumed that NK cells express p75 and that binding to this molecule provides the stimulus for proliferation. However, confirmation of this hypothesis depends on the (eagerly awaited) development of a monoclonal antibody to this protein.

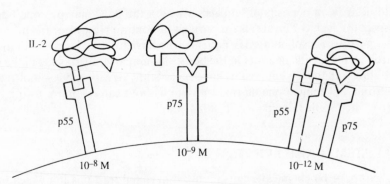

Fig. 5.6 The two chain IL-2–R. The high-affinity IL-2 receptor consists of two polypeptide chains with differing binding affinities. The p55 (Tac) protein is found in excess of p75 on stimulated T-cells whereas the p75 is found on NK cells which do not have the Tac protein.

IL-2 receptor expression and adult T-cell leukaemia

In recent years, abnormally high levels of the Tac molecule has been found on the surface of fresh or cultured leukaemic cells derived from patients with adult T-cell leukaemia (ATL) (Depper *et al.*, 1984). ATL is an aggressive virus-induced leukaemia, which is prevalent in several countries including parts of Japan, the Caribbean, the USA and Africa. The leukaemia results from infection with an oncogenic (tumour-producing) retrovirus known as human T-cell lymphotropic virus (HTLV) I. HTLV-I infects CD4$^+$ cells (helper T-cells), where the viral RNA is transcribed into DNA by its reverse transcriptase enzyme. The viral DNA integrates into the host genome where replication is initiated by products of the viral 'transactivating transcriptional element' (*tat*) gene. Cell lines derived from HTLV-I-infected T-cells have been shown to bind over 300 000 molecules of Anti-Tac, roughly ten times the number which is found on PHA-stimulated T-cells. The majority of these receptors bind IL-2 with low affinity and indeed some cells lines have no high-affinity receptors whatsoever. The significance of the large number of Tac molecules on ATL cells is not fully understood. Continued growth of these cells in culture does not depend on exogenous IL-2 although it is possible that endogenous IL-2 stimulates their growth, or even further release of IL-2, in an autocrine fashion. The binding of IL-2 to activated, non-infected T-cells is known to result in an increased expression of the Tac protein. It is possible that the virus encodes a factor which induces the gene for the Tac protein and one such canditate is the product of the *tat* gene (Green and Leonard, 1986).

Whatever the mechanism involved, the presence of high levels of IL-2 receptor on ATL cells has opened up prospects for therapy with Anti-Tac conjugated to toxins. Several recent studies have demonstrated that conjugates of Anti-Tac to purified ricin A chain markedly inhibit the growth of ATL cells *in vitro*. Although it is hard to see how administration of such conjugates to patients with ATL could destroy all deposits of leukaemia within the bone marrow, one hopeful prospect for such conjugates is for purging of bone marrow prior to autologous bone-marrow transplantation in patients who have received lethal irradiation to destroy all leukaemic deposits in the body. Preliminary experiments in the USA have shown that such conjugates have successfully destroyed 99.9% of tumour cells from leukaemic bone marrow *in vitro* without causing harm to the bone-marrow stem cells (Kronke *et al.*, 1984).

CELL-MEMBRANE EVENTS

The nature of biochemical events involved in signal transmission which follow the binding of IL-2 to high-affinity receptors is still uncertain. The finding that the cytoplasmic portion of the Tac molecule was so small, raised doubts about its ability to transmit a signal across the cell membrane. These doubts were allayed by the discovery of p75, which has a much larger anchorage peptide. When radiolabelled IL-2 binds to high-affinity receptors, it becomes internalized following receptor-mediated endocytosis. The half-life for cell-bound IL-2 is 25–30 min. Nonetheless, the following biochemical activities have been shown to be increased after high-affinity binding, although the individual involvement of each is not fully appreciated:

(1) Stimulation of phosphoinositol turnover: IL-2 rapidly stimulates the hydrolysis of phosphoinositides in an IL-2-dependent murine cytotoxic T-cell line. Such breakdown of membrane phospholipids has frequently been found to act as a membrane transduction mechanism in other receptor/ligand signalling where interaction at the cell surface stimulates phospholipase C which hydrolyses phosphatidylinositol biphosphate to acylglycerol and inositol triphosphate.

(2) IL-2 stimulates redistribution of protein kinase C (PK-C) from the cytoplasm to the cell membrane. PK-C is again part of a common membrane transduction mechanism. Diacylglycerol produced by phosphoinositol hydrolysis activates PK-C which is then translocated to the membrane where it catalyses the ATP-dependent phosphorylation of several protein substrates. Similarly, inositol triphosphate stimulates the release of Ca^{2+} from intracellular stores which in turn can activate Ca^{2+}-dependent kinases such as PK-C.

(3) IL-2 has been shown to modulate membrane adenylate cyclase activity and to stimulate GTPase activity of isolated membranes.

(4) Binding of IL-2 to cell surface receptors stimulates the IL-2 receptor gene resulting in an increased expression of IL-2 receptors, with low-affinity receptors being preferentially increased (Smith and Cantrell, 1985). Activation of the *tac* protein gene can be demonstrated within 3 h of IL-2 binding and reaches a peak within 24 h. Activation of other genes also occurs and in particular there is sequential activation of the genes for IFN-γ,

IL-2 itself and (later) genes for the transferrin receptor. Transferrin is required by all growing cells and its binding to cell surface receptors precedes the transfer from the G_1 phase of the cell cycle to the S phase.

Clinical use for IL-2

Much interest has been generated recently by the use of IL-2 in cancer therapy, as can be judged by the number of 'popular science' TV and radio programmes which have featured this lymphokine and by the increasing price of shares in biotechnology firms which make recombinant human IL-2. In addition to its potential as an anticancer drug, it has been administered to patients suffering immunodeficiency disease, in attempts to replace some immunological reactivity.

IMMUNOTHERAPY OF CANCER

There are several lines of evidence which suggest that tumours express novel antigenic determinants not present on the corresponding normal tissue. Moreover, there is also evidence that many patients do mount an immune response (albeit an inadequate one) against their tumour and that this can be measured *in vitro* (Dawson and Moore, 1989). For example, T-cells isolated from the blood of tumour-bearing patients can sometimes be shown to be cytotoxic towards cells derived from their own tumour (that is, autologous) although rarely are they cytotoxic towards allogeneic tumours, even those of similar type. When unfixed sections of tumours are stained immunohistologically, using specific monoclonal antibodies, they are frequently found to be infiltrated by lymphocytes and monocytes although the degree of infiltration is seldom correlated with prognosis in humans. Lymphocytes have been isolated from these tumour infiltrates, cloned, and shown to be cytotoxic to cells of the fresh tumour. Such lymphocytes are considered to be a better indicator of antitumour immunity than lymphocytes obtained from peripheral blood. One point of view suggests that the development of a tumour in a patient represents a failure of the immune response to recognize tumour cells as foreign. In support of this theory, patients with a large tumour frequently fail to respond to a variety of 'common' immunogens to which they might be expected to be immunized. Tumour products can themselves be immunosuppressive, but the consequences may not be recognized until the tumour reaches a critical size. Added to this, some chemotherapeutic agents may also strongly inhibit the production of IL-2 and thus contribute to the underlying immunodeficiency. Numerous attempts have been made to boost the general immune response of cancer-bearing patients with immunomodulatory substances, the best-known examples being Bacillus Calmette-Guérin (BCG) which stimulates the tumoricidal activity of macrophages, and interferon which also has growth-inhibitory properties. Both of these biological response modifiers have had limited success with tumours despite extensive trials over some years.

Recently, attention has centred on the use of IL-2 to promote the differentiation of lymphokine-activated killer cells (LAK) (Rosenberg, 1985). Lymphocyte populations obtained from healthy or tumour-bearing individuals are rarely cytotoxic *in vitro* towards cells obtained from fresh human tumours. However, after culturing the lymphocytes for 48 h with IL-2, they develop a cytotoxicity towards a variety of tumours derived from different tissues, including melanomas, sarcomas and carcinomas. Normal tissue is resistant to lysis by LAK cells. The cytotoxicity which can be induced in lymphocyte populations by prolonged incubation in IL-2 is not associated with the small lymphocyte population but with larger (LAK) cells bearing cell surface markers similar to cytotoxic T-lymphocytes, but without the specificity of the latter. LAK therapy involves the infusion into cancer patients of their own (autologous) lymphocytes which have been activated *in vitro* with IL-2 for a minimum of 48 h. The efficacy of this approach was first demonstrated in an animal model: when mice are injected with syngeneic melanoma cells intravenously, melanoma cells develop into tumour nodules within the lungs. When such mice were injected with spleen cells which had been cultured in IL-2 for several days, there was a significant decrease in the number of established tumour nodules, i.e. LAK treatment had caused regression of some of the tumour nodules (Mazumder and Rosenberg, 1984).

IL-2 has been tested for antitumour effects in cancer patients either on its own, or as part of LAK therapy, in several trials world-wide. The testing of new treatments for human disease is carried out in stages, where each stage has a specific aim. Phase 1 trials serve to establish the toxicity of any drug or treatment, and to provide information on the pharmacokinetics. The aim is to determine maximum tolerated doses and the best routes of administration and timing of doses. In Phase 2 trials, information obtained from Phase 1 is used to establish the efficacy of the drug in the clinical situation. The latter is usually carried out with 'double-blind' trials in which all patients are coded and entered at random into two treatment groups: those patients receiving conventional treatment and those receiving the experimental treatment. At the end of the trial, the patient codes are deciphered and the effects of the treatments analysed. Of course, if, during the course of a phase 2 trial one treatment group is demonstrably faring either much better or worse than the other, it is essential to stop the trials and put all patients onto the 'better' treatment. Phase 1 and 2 trials have been conducted with IL-2 or LAK therapy being administered to cancer patients, and the results are summarized below (Rosenberg *et al.*, 1985).

Phase 1

Interleukin-2 has been administered either by a series of individual (bolus) injections, or by intravenous infusion for several hours. Doses administered in various studies have ranged from 10^3 to 10^6 U/m^2 of body area or from 10^4 to 10^5 U/kg body weight. When IL-2 is injected intravenously it is rapidly cleared from the blood. The plasma half-life, which has been estimated at 5–7 min, can only be minimally increased by subcutaneous or intraperitoneal injections. The rapid clearance of exogenous IL-2, brought about by renal catabolism, coupled possibly with plasma inhibitors, has important consequences for cancer therapy based on the ability of IL-2 to stimulate the LAK precursor. The production of LAK cells involves direct interaction between the precursors and the IL-2 which may not happen when the half-life is so short – hence the need to activate the cells *in vitro*. Attempts have been made to circumvent this rapid clearance by administering IL-2 by different routes. For example, in cancer patients it may be more beneficial to administer the lymphokine directly into an artery serving the site of a primary tumour, although where there are metastases, this is more of a problem. Delivering the drug in phospholipid liposomes may prolong the half-life of the molecule and this has been successful for other lymphokines. Another method currently under trial is to inject IL-2 directly into the splenic artery. LAK precursors are found in the spleen and these are more likely to be activated if a comparatively high local dose can be achieved. Alternatively, multiple repeated bolus injections each day would be needed to maintain continuous high levels in the blood and, given the current price of recombinant lymphokines, the cost might prove to be prohibitively expensive.

The toxicity of treatment with IL-2 depends very much on the type of therapeutic approach used, the most toxic effects occurring during LAK therapy in which patients may receive several doses of IL-2 together with LAK cells produced by activation of patients' lymphocytes *in vitro*. A protocol for LAK therapy is shown in Fig. 5.7. The administration of IL-2 alone results in an initial, rapid decline in the circulating white cell count although the numbers return to normal within 24 h. Large numbers of eosinophils are frequently found in the blood. The mechanism of this eosinophilia is unclear although it may be related to the release of IL-5, a lymphokine which stimulates the growth and differentiation of eosinophils from stem cells in the bone marrow (see Chapter 7). Up to 2 mg of natural IL-2 could be safely infused into cancer patients. The most frequent adverse reactions associated with administration of natural or recombinant IL-2 include fever, chills, fatigue, malaise, nausea and vomiting. In addition, leakage of capillaries leads to fluid retention and sudden, excessive weight gains. One or more of these symptoms occur in approximately 25% of patients undergoing IL-2 therapy, the greatest toxicity being associated with administration of LAK cells, where toxicity is rapidly manifested after infusion of LAK. Some symptoms, such as fever, chills, nausea and vomiting can to some extent be controlled with drugs, but fluid retention is seen as a very serious problem, causing oedema, respiratory distress, hypotension, and acute renal failure. Severe fluid retention may necessitate the discontinuation of LAK therapy since it can result in the death of the patient. These toxic effects cannot be ignored and currently the mortality associated with treatment with LAK cells and IL-2 is around 2%.

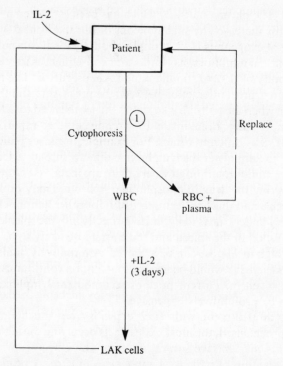

Fig. 5.7 Protocol for LAK therapy. Cytophoresis is a process in which blood is removed from the patient, fractionated by centrifugation, and the unwanted fractions returned to the patient. In this case, the white-cell population is retained and the red cells and plasma returned (1). The white cells are incubated with IL-2 for a minimum of 48 h and returned to the patient together with more IL-2. A LAK therapy may involve several cytophoreses, possibly on successive days.

Efficacy

The results of several trials with LAK therapy are now available (Rosenberg *et al.*, 1985; Fagan and Eddleston, 1987). In most cases reported, only the administration of IL-2 together with LAK cells has proved to be effective although it is becoming apparent that very high doses of IL-2 may be as effective as LAK cells in causing tumour regression. In at least one study, patients have generally been shown to tolerate multiple cell infusions of 2×10^{11} autologous LAK cells and an objective regression of tumours, that is, $> 50\%$ reduction of tumour volume, has been demonstrated in a significant number of cancer patients with tumours of a variety of histogenic origins. Moreover, attempts have been made to administer autologous LAK cells, expanded *in vitro* in IL-2, by injection into the tumour foci of melanoma and breast cancer lesions. Partial regressions of individual lesions were seen in several cases. Such an approach is not, however, very practical, since metastasized lesions may be inaccessible even to surgery. Similarly, the protocols for LAK therapy are logistically very difficult, involving as they do several plasmaphoreses to remove blood, and multiple injections of activated LAK cells which result from several days' incubation.

The most extensive clinical trials for LAK therapy have been carried out at the National Cancer Institute in Bethesda where over 200 patients with advanced cancer have now been treated. Partial regression of tumours had been seen in a number of patients, 16 of whom experienced complete regression of their tumour. The tumours which are most sensitive to LAK cells are renal cell carcinomas, malignant melanomas, colorectal carcinomas and non-Hodgkin's lymphoma. Unfortunately, LAK therapy appears to be ineffective against the most common tumours such as those of the lung or the breast. The development of new treatments, especially for cancer, always presents dilemmas, particularly if the results are not overwhelmingly successful and if the treatment itself is highly toxic. It must also be recognized that the majority of patients so far treated by LAK therapy have been patients with advanced cancer for whom conventional radiotherapy and chemotherapy have failed. People with advanced cancer are much more likely to be susceptible to the toxicity of any treatment, including further chemotherapy. Variations on LAK therapy are being tried out in order to increase the 'success rate' of this treatment. For example, the use of animal models has demonstrated that tumour-infiltrating lymphocytes may be more effective at killing tumours than LAK cells. In addition, other lymphokines, or even cocktails of lymphokines, may prove to be more effective activators of cytotoxic cells *in vivo*.

IL-2 AND IMMUNE REPLACEMENT THERAPY

Patients who, for whatever reason, are deficient in helper T-cells, will consequently be deficient in the lymphokines that they produce and, since IL-2 is a central molecule in the development of an effective immune response, it is possible that exogenous IL-2 might replace some of the functions missing in these individuals. Although congenital immunodeficiency affecting T-cells is rare, the incidence of acquired immunodeficiency resulting from infection with the human immunodeficiency virus (HIV) is increasing at an alarming rate and it is here that most replacement therapy has been attempted.

HUMAN IMMUNODEFICIENCY VIRUS AND AIDS

The human immunodeficiency virus (HIV) is a retrovirus (Fig. 5.8) which also infects cells expressing the CD4 cell surface molecule, the majority of which are the helper T-lymphocytes. HIV has been classified as a member of the lentivirus group of retroviruses. These viruses all cause slow, protracted wasting diseases. After infection of cells the virus may remain quiescent within the cell with or without integration into the genome (see *Scientific American*, 1988). When HIV

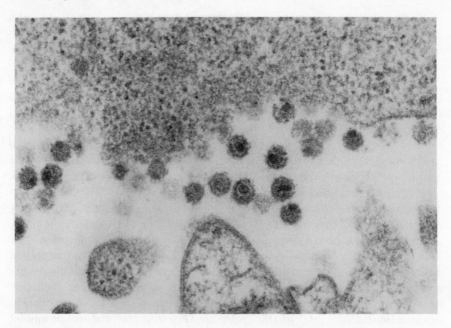

Fig. 5.8   The HIV virus. The electron micrograph shows whole viral particles emerging from an infected lymphoblastoid cell line. Magnification × 92 000. (Courtesy of Alan Curry, Public Health Laboratory, Withington Hospital, Manchester.)

becomes integrated into the genome of the helper T-lymphocyte, activation of that cell during the process of a normal immune response results in concomitant activation of the virus, which replicates and causes lysis of the host cell. Patients infected with HIV, and especially if they have AIDS, frequently have reduced numbers of helper T-cells and the CD4:CD8 ratio may be as low as 0.5:1 instead of the usual 2:1. Consequently, while potential effector cells (B-cells and Tc) are present and can respond to antigen by elaboration of IL-2 receptors, very little IL-2 (as well as numerous other lymphokines) is available to support their growth and differentiation. Thus, opportunistic infections, typically those listed in Table 5.1, are a common cause of death in these patients. Similarly, patients with AIDS or the AIDS-related complex which precedes the full-blown disease, fail to exhibit skin reactions to a panel of common antigens such as mumps, PPD, *Candida* and tetanus toxoid, to which they might reasonably be expected to be immune. Patients with AIDS also commonly suffer from a particularly aggressive form of Kaposi's sarcoma, a tumour of vascular tissue origin which appears as red nodules in the skin, mouth, gut and lungs. This usually rare tumour may be related to infection with cytomegalovirus (CMV), a ubiquitous virus which is frequently reactivated in these patients. Similarly, about 5% of

Table 5.1 Opportunistic infection in the diagnosis of AIDS

Viral	Bacterial	Fungal	Protozoal and helminthic
Cytomegalovirus	Atypical mycobacteria	Candidosis	*Pneumocystis carinii* pneumonia
		Histoplasmosis	Toxoplasmosis
Herpes simplex		Cryptococcosis	Cryptosporidiosis
		Isosporiasis	Strongyloidosis

patients with AIDS develop non-Hodgkin's lymphomas which may be associated with infection with the Epstein–Barr (EB) virus.

The only treatments so far available for patients with AIDS are aimed either at treating the opportunistic infection, for example with antibiotics, or using drugs such as azidothymidine (AZT) aimed at inhibiting viral replication. While control of the spread of the disease is dependent on an effective combination of antiviral therapy and vaccination, as yet no drug is capable of completely eradicating the virus and the development and testing of vaccines may take several years. The failure to deal specifically with infectious agents, and the inactivity of NK cells towards virus-infected cells can be attributed to low lymphokine levels in these patients. Since patients who develop the full-blown AIDS invariably die from opportunistic infection and since the incidence of infection with the virus is increasing dramatically, there is need of a therapy to support their ailing immune system at least until such time as curative treatments are available.

IL-2 replacement in AIDS

When lymphocytes from AIDS patients are incubated *in vitro* with IL-2, virus-specific cytotoxic T-lymphocytes are found in the cultures, indicating the presence of precursors with IL-2R in these patients (Sheridan *et al.*, 1984). Similarly, IL-2 can restore an almost total loss of NK activity *in vitro*. Administration of IL-2 to these patients can restore some of their immune deficit when measured in conventional NK assays or by skin testing with panels of common immunogens. Whereas the total number of CD4$^+$ cells does not increase significantly following IL-2 treatment, decreases in the CD8 levels have resulted in an increase in the CD4$^+$:CD8$^+$ ratios. Detectable serum levels of IL-2 in these patients has only been seen following bolus injection of 25×10^4 units. In one trial, no patient developed new infections during the course of treatment with IL-2 and other patients recovered from the severe diarrhoea which is caused by cryptosporidial infection. Individual lesions of Kaposi's sarcoma have been shown to become sharply demarcated in treated patients and some have shown minor regression although in no case has total regression been demonstrated (Kern *et al.*, 1985; Volberding *et al.*, 1985). On the whole, the effects of IL-2 in these patients have been inconsistent and disappointing and this may reflect the fact that a normal immune response involves a 'cocktail' of lymphokines which act synergistically. Successful immune replacement with lymphokines requires much more knowledge concerning the interaction of different molecules as well as greater availability of the gene-cloned products. However, even with an extensive knowledge of lymphokine biology, the fact remains that the origin of this syndrome is viral and, so long as the virus remains in the body, then treatment with lymphokines will bring temporary relief only. The only effective ways of dealing with the global AIDS epidemic are prevention and the development of successful non-toxic antiviral drugs. The most likely preventive measure, apart from changes in lifestyle, will be immunization against HIV. Many laboratories world-wide are working on the design and development of HIV vaccines and there are already reports of at least one vaccine which is ready for testing by individuals in high-risk groups.

Summary

Interleukin-2 is a central molecule of the immune response, being absolutely essential for the proliferation and differentiation of antigen-exposed B- and T-lymphocytes. It also appears to trigger the release of other lymphokines from helper T-cells. IL-2 also has important effects on NK and LAK cells and may for this reason be important in non-specific immunity towards tumour cells and virus-infected cells. Although much is already known about the nature of the active molecule and about the cell surface receptors to which it binds, little is known about the nature of signal transmission following binding. Much interest has been recently generated by the use of IL-2 in cancer therapy where its use has been associated with complete tumour regression, in particular, of renal cell carcinomas and malignant melanomas. Unfortunately, the treatment has also been associated with the death of just over 2% of cancer patients who are treated with LAK therapy. IL-2 has also been used to treat patients with AIDS, where it can reduce the number of opportunistic infections which are experienced. Finally, it must not be forgotten that the ability of IL-2 to promote the growth of T-lymphocytes in culture has been invaluable in increasing our knowledge of the very cells themselves.

References

Aarden, L. A., Brunner, T. K. and Cerotinni, J.-C. *et al.* (1979). 'Revised nomenclature for antigen non-specific T cell proliferation and helper factors', *J. Immunol.* **123**, p. 2928.

Cantrell, D. A. and Smith, K. A. (1983). 'Transient expression of interleukin-2 receptors', *J. Exp. Med.* **158**, p. 1895.

Clark, S. C. and Kamen, R. (1987). 'The human haemopoietic colony-stimulating factors', *Science* **236**, p. 1229.

Dawson M. M. and Moore, M. (1989). 'Immunity to tumours' in *Immunology*, 2nd edn, Eds Roitt, I., Brostoff, J. and Male, D. London, Gower Medical Publishing.

Depper, J. M., Leonard, W. J., Kronke, M., Waldmann, T. A. and Greene, W. C. (1984). 'Augmented T cell growth factor receptor expression in HTLV-I-infected human leukaemic cells', *J. Immunol.* **133**, p. 1691.

Fagan, E. A. and Eddleston, A. L. W. (1987). 'Immunotherapy for cancer: the use of lymphokine-activated killer (LAK) cells', *Gut* **28**, p. 113.

Greene, W. C. and Leonard, W. J. (1986). 'The human interleukin-2 receptor', *Ann. Rev. Immunol.* **4**, p. 69.

Greene, W. C. and Robb, R. J. (1985). 'Receptors for T-cell growth factor: structure, function and expression on normal and neoplastic cells' in *Contemporary Topics in Molecular Biology*, Vol. 10, *The Interleukins*. London, Plenum Press.

Grimm, E. A., Mazumder, A., Zhang, H. Z. and Rosenberg, S. A. (1982). 'Lymphokine-activated killer cell phenomenon. Lysis of natural killer-resistant fresh solid tumour cells by interleukin-2-activated autologous human peripheral blood lymphocytes', *J. Exp. Med.* **155**, p. 1823.

Kern, P., Toy, J. and Dietrich, M. (1985). 'Preliminary clinical observations with recombinant interleukin-2 in patients with AIDS or LAS', *Blut* **50**, p. 1.

Kohler, G. and Milstein, C. (1975). 'Continuous cultures of fused cells secreting antibody of predefined specificity', *Nature (London)* **256**, p. 495.

Kronke, M., Depper, J. M., Leonard, W. J., Vitetta, E. S., Waldmann, T. A. and Greene, W. C. (1984). 'Human T cell leukaemia/lymphoma virus-infected leukaemic T cells are selectively killed by anti-T cell growth factor receptor immunotoxins', *Clin. Res.* **32**, p. 418.

Malkowsky, M. and Medawar, P. B. (1984). 'Is immunological tolerance (non-responsiveness) a consequence of interleukin-2 deficit during the recognition of antigen?', *Immunol. Today* **5**, p. 340.

Mazumder, A. and Rosenberg, S. A. (1984). 'Successful immunotherapy of natural killer-resistant established pulmonary melanoma metastases by the intravenous adoptive transfer of syngeneic lymphocytes activated *in vitro* by interleukin 2', *J. Exp. Med.* **159**, p. 495.

Meidema, F. and Melief, J. M. (1985). 'T cell regulation of human B-cell activation. A reappraisal of the role of interleukin-2', *Immunol. Today* **6**, p. 258.

Morgan, D. A., Ruscetti, F. W. and Gallo, R. (1976). 'Selective *in vivo* growth of T lymphocytes from normal human bone marrows', *Science* **193**, p. 1007.

Mosmann, T. R. and Coffman, R. L. (1987). 'Two types of mouse helper T cell clone – implications for immune regulations', *Immunol. Today* **8**, p. 223.

Robb, R. J. (1984). 'Interleukin-2: the molecule and its function', *Immunol. Today* **5**, p. 203.

Robb, R., Kutny, R. M., Panico, M. *et al.* (1984). 'Amino acid sequence and post-translational modification of human interleukin-2'. *Proc. Natl Acad. Sci. (USA)* **81**, p. 6486.

Rosenberg, S. A. (1985). 'Lymphokine-activated killer cells: a new approach to immunotherapy of cancer', *J. Natl Cancer Inst.* **75**, p. 595.

Rosenberg, S. A. (1988). 'Immunotherapy of cancer using interleukin-2: current status and future prospects', *Immunol. Today* **9**, p. 58.

Rosenberg, S. A., Lotz, M. T., Muul, L. M. *et al.* (1985). 'Observations on the systemic administration of autologous lymphokine-activated killer cells and recombinant interleukin-2 to patients with metastatic cancer'. *New Engl J. Med.* **313**, p. 1485.

Scientific American (1988). 'What science knows about AIDS', **259**.

Sheridan, J. F., Aurelian, L. and Quinn, T. C. (1984). 'Modulation of virus-specific immunity *in vitro* by the addition of interleukin-1 and interleukin-2 in patients with the acquired immune deficiency syndrome', *Ann. NY Acad. Sci.* **437**, p. 530.

Smith, K. A. (1987). 'The two-chain structure of high affinity IL-2 receptors', *Immunol. Today* **8**, p. 11.

Smith, K. and Cantrell, D. (1985). 'Interleukin-2 regulates its own receptors', *Proc. Natl Acad. Sci. (USA)* **82**, p. 864.

Taniguchi, T., Matsui, H., Fujita, T. *et al.* (1983). 'Structure and expression of a cloned cDNA for human interleukin-2', *Nature (London)* **302**, p. 305.

Trinchieri, G., Matsumoto-Kobayashi, M., Clark, S. C. *et al.* (1984). 'Response of resting human peripheral blood NK cells to IL-2', *J. Exp. Med.* **16**, p. 1147.

Uchiyama, T., Broder, S. and Waldmann, T. A. (1981). 'A monoclonal antibody (Anti-Tac) reactive with activated and functionally mature human T cells. I. production of Anti-Tac monoclonal antibody and distribution of Tac (+) cells', *J. Immunol.* **126**. p. 1393.

Volberding, P. A., Wofsy, C. B. and Abrams, D. I. (1985). 'Interferon and interleukin-2 therapy of Kaposi's sarcoma', *Adv. Exp. Med. Biol.* **18**, p. 151.

6

Interleukin-3

Introduction

Interleukin-3 (IL-3) is a haemopoietic growth factor, i.e. a protein which regulates the number of cells in the blood by promoting the division of the stem cells in the bone marrow. Like other 'haemopoietins', IL-3 also promotes the differentiation of the progeny of the stem cells. Il-3 can influence the production of a range of leukocytes including all three groups of polymorphonuclear leukocyte, monocytes, erythrocytes and megakaryocytes, which gives rise to the blood platelets. For this reason, IL-3 is sometimes known as a 'panhaemopoietin' (*pan* is Greek for 'all'). IL-3 is also a growth factor for mast cells which, though not found in the blood, also originate from stem cells in the bone marrow. Although numerous other haemopoietins exist, these are not produced by lymphocytes or have as their main site of production, non-lymphocytic cells. For this reason, this chapter will concentrate on IL-3. However, mention will also be made of the uses of a somewhat similar molecule, GM-CSF (granulocyte–macrophage colony stimulating factor) which is also produced by lymphocytes (though not exclusively) and which has been the subject of a number of clinical trials in recent years. Mention should also be made at this point of the newly characterized interleukin-7 (IL-7), which is the product of stromal cells within the bone marrow and which acts principally to stimulate the production of B-lymphocytes within the bone marrow. This molecule will be discussed in Chapter 7 which deals with factors affecting B-lymphocytes.

Interleukin-3

Although IL-3 is concerned principally with haemopoiesis, the name was assigned on the basis of a quite distinct activity, namely, the induction of an enzyme involved in progesterone metabolism (Ihle *et al.*, 1981), a somewhat esoteric activity which is, nonetheless, of immunological significance. Later, the molecule was shown to encompass numerous activities which had been described several years earlier. Thus, the molecules listed in Table 6.1 can now be considered as alternative names for IL-3. While these names are interchangeable, for reasons of clarity the term IL-3 will be used wherever possible. The evidence that IL-3 mediates all these activities is extensive. It has, for example, proved impossible, by whatever purification procedure used, to separate the different activities from each other (Ihle *et al.*, 1983). In addition, recombinant IL-3 has been shown to mediate all of these activities. The ability of IL-3 to mediate effects on a variety of cell types reflects an increasingly familiar phenomenon. Indeed, such multiple activities could now be written into the 'job-description' of such molecules. The discovery of a new factor which affects haemopoiesis, and which has multiple effects on different blood cell types was, and remains, an exciting prospect. IL-3 was first reported in mice and the vast majority of research work on it has been performed on this species, hence the inevitable bias in this chapter towards the murine form. However, human IL-3 has more recently been discovered and the gene cloned (Yang *et al.*, 1986) and this, and other haemopoietic growth factors, may be of use in restoring full bone-marrow activity in patients whose own marrow has been depleted, for example by accidental or therapeutic irradiation or by toxic drugs such as those used for cancer chemotherapy.

Table 6.1   Alternative names for interleukin-3

Name	Activity promoted
Multi-CSF (colony stimulating factor)	Growth of haemopoietic stem cells
Panspecific haemopoietin (PSH)	Growth of haemopoietic stem cells
P-cell stimulating factor	Growth of mast cells from spleen cultures
WEHI-3B factor*	Long-term growth of bone-marrow cultures
Burst promoting activity	Growth of erythroid colonies from bone marrow
Mast-cell growth factor	Proliferation of mast cells in cultures of spleen and bone marrow
CFU (colony-forming unit) stimulating factor	Growth of haemopoietic stem cells
Histamine-producing cell stimulating factor	Growth and maturation of mast cells

*WEHI-3B is a cell line derived from a murine leukaemia which produces IL-3 constitutively. The leukaemia is classified as myelomonocytic although the cells also express Thy-1, a glycoprotein expressed on murine T-cells.

The precise cellular source of IL-3 has been examined by several approaches including the cloning of activated T-lymphocytes and the production of T-cell hybridomas. Similarly, cell lines from T-cell lymphomas have also been activated with mitogen and the supernatants examined for IL-3 activity. These separate approaches have both confirmed that the helper T-lymphocyte is the chief producer of IL-3 as measured either by the induction of 20α-hydroxysteroid dehydrogenase (20αSDH) in *nu/nu* spleen cells, or by the ability to support the growth of IL-3 dependent cell lines. IL-3 is produced by cells which concomitantly release multiple lymphokine activities including IL-2 and IFN-γ. In mice, where two types of helper T-cells (T_{H1} and T_{H2}) have been cloned, both types have been shown to produce IL-3. T_{H1} also produce IFN-γ and IL-2 whereas T_{H2} are known to produce IL-4 and IL-5 (Mosmann and Coffman, 1987).

INTERLEUKIN-3 AND THE INDUCTION OF 20α-HYDROXYSTEROID DEHYDROGENASE (20αSDH)

The enzyme 20αSDH catalyses the reduction of progesterone to 20α-dihydroprogesterone (20αOHP) using reducing power from NADPH. Its activity can be measured by monitoring the conversion of radiolabelled progesterone to radiolabelled 20αOHP. 20αSDH has for some time been used as a marker for mature T-lymphocytes so that its induction could indicate differentiation in T-cell precursors. The evidence for this association comes from several sources and includes the following:

(1) Studies of the distribution of 20αSDH (Table 6.2) which revealed that it is absent from immature lymphoid tissues and from lymphoid tissues obtained from athymic mice. Mice can be rendered athymic if the thymus is

Table 6.2 Location of 20αSDH activity

Tissue/cells	20αSDH*
Spleen cells	+ +
T-depleted spleen cells	±
nu/nu spleen cells	±
Spleen cells from neonatally thymectomized animals	±
B-cells	±
B-cells lines	±
Macrophage lines	±
Helper T-cell lines	+
Cytotoxic T-cell lines	+ + +
nu/nu spleen cells + Con-A conditioned medium	+ + +

*Activities: + + +, high; + +, medium; +, low; ±, negligible

removed during the critical neonatal period. Such mice have no mature T-cells which is assumed to be due to an inability to 'seed' the secondary lymphoid organs with mature T-cells in the neonatal period. In addition, there is an inbred strain of mice (*nu/nu* mice) which have no thymus, so that T-cells are never processed during fetal life. Lymphocytes obtained from both neonatally thymectomized and *nu/nu* mice have very low levels of 20αSDH activity.

(2) In normal adult mice 20αSDH is only found in mature T-cells which are easily identified because they express Thy-1, an integral membrane glycoprotein. If mature T-cells are removed from a lymphocyte population, by incubating the cells with an antibody to Thy-1 and fresh complement, the 20αSDH activity is significantly reduced.

IL-3 was discovered during attempts to identify molecules which could induce T-cells to differentiate in spleen cells from *nu/nu* mice, using the expression of 20αSDH to indicate T-cell maturation. During these experiments, a factor in the conditioned media from Con-A-stimulated mouse lymphocytes was found to be a potent inducer of 20αSDH after only 6 h incubation (Fig. 6.1). This result suggested that precursors for T-lymphocytes are present in the spleens of *nu/nu* mice but that they lack a differentiation factor. However, complete maturation of T-cells, that is, to

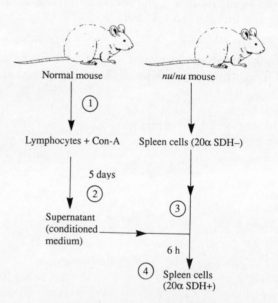

Fig. 6.1 Induction of 20αSDH by Con-A-conditioned medium. Spleen cells removed from a normal mouse and activated with Con-A (1), release lymphokines into the medium (2). When this medium is incubated with 20αSDH-deficient spleen cells from athymic mice, (3) these cells become 20αSDH-positive after 6 h incubation (4).

cells expressing the Thy-1 antigen, could not be induced in athymic mice. The active factor in Con-A supernatants was extensively purified and characterized, shown to be unrelated to any of the unknown lymphokines, including IL-2 and named IL-3 (Ihle, 1985).

Is 20αSDH a marker for T-lymphocytes?

The view that the enzyme 20αSDH is unique to T-lymphocytes, or even that it may be used as a marker of T-cell differentiation, has been the subject of much lively debate. The objections can be summarized as follows:

(1) 20αSDH is not, after all, exclusive to T-lymphocytes and is found in several cell types including polymorphonuclear leukocytes, mast cells and tumour cells of mast cell origin (Garland and Dexter, 1982; Hapel *et al.*, 1985). Thus the induction of the enzyme in *nu/nu* spleen cells may represent its induction in mast cells or PMN precursors rather than T-cells. Since T-cells are the main producers of IL-3, it is not surprising that athymic mice are deficient in 20αSDH. Similarly, any treatment which depletes spleen cells of T-lymphocytes will remove the source of IL-3 and result in lowered activity of 20αSDH, *but not necessarily in T-cells.*

(2) Other factors which stimulate haemopoiesis have been reported to increase 20αSDH in bone-marrow cultures. In fact, the enzyme might be more properly regarded as an indicator of proliferating haemopoietic tissue rather than of T-cell maturation.

Whatever, the outcome of this debate, the induction of 20αSDH in populations of spleen cells from athymic mice still provides a means for the bioassay of IL-3 and for monitoring the progress of its purification from conditioned media. There is little doubt, though that the importance of IL-3 lies in its ability to stimulate the division and differentiation of haemopoietic stem cells. IL-3 is unique in having effects on most of the formed elements of the blood and is also involved in the production and differentiation of mast cells.

INTERLEUKIN-3 AND HAEMOPOIESIS

The cells in the blood have a variable life-span depending on the histological type. Most blood cells, with the exception of some small lymphocytes, are short-lived and survive in the circulation for a matter of days or weeks. Despite this fairly rapid turnover of cells, numbers of cells in the blood remains fairly stable in a healthy individual and this is because dead cells are removed from the circulation and replaced by new cells derived from division of stem cells within the haemopoietic tissues. The major source of haemopoietic tissue in an adult animal is the bone marrow although smaller 'pockets' also occur in the lymph nodes, spleen and thymus.

Investigation of haemopoietic stem cells: colony-forming units

The different lineages of cells in the blood are all derived ultimately from the same stem cells which are therefore said to be pluripotential. The stem cells give rise, by mitosis, to undifferentiated cells that are capable, at the time of their production, of differentiating into any of the white blood cells including megakaryocytes. Even at this stage, the daughter cells may become stem cells, giving rise to cells

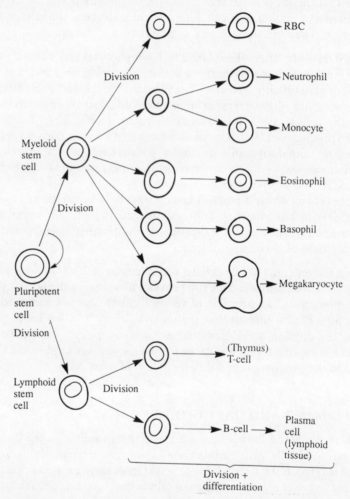

Fig. 6.2 The haemopoietic pathway. The pluripotent stem cell in the bone marrow divides and gives rise to the lymphoid stem cell, from which arise the B- and T-lymphocytes, and the myeloid from which all other formed elements of the blood are derived, including the platelets. All stem cells are capable of self-renewal as well as providing undifferentiated cells which will differentiate into blood cells.

with restricted potential for development. Along the haemopoietic pathway (Fig. 6.2) we can see that cells become channelled into different pathways of development (Weiss, 1984). Haemopoietic stem cells can be investigated in animals by one of at least two means:

Spleen colony assay. The spleen colony assay, illustrated in Fig. 6.3, relies on the ability of freshly isolated bone-marrow cells to re-populate the spleens of lethally irradiated mice. Several days after the intravenous injection of bone-marrow cells, the spleens of injected mice have a nodular appearance where each nodule represents a colony produced from a stem cell. When individual colonies are examined histologically, some are found to contain a number of blood cell types whereas others may contain a single, or perhaps two, cell types. The former are derived from the uncommitted or pluripotent stem cell, and are therefore called CFU-S (colony forming unit, spleen). The second type of colony, which contains a single or at the most two cell types, represents the product of a stem

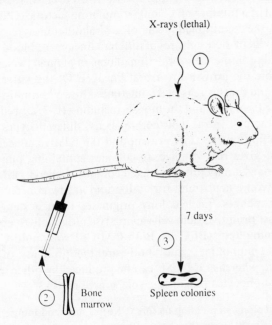

Fig. 6.3 The spleen colony assay. Irradiation of mice with sufficiently high doses of X-rays destroys the haemopoietic stem cells in the bone marrow (1). These mice can be restored with bone marrow from syngeneic animals (2). The stem cells in the injected bone marrow populate the spleen and each stem cell gives rise to a colony in the spleen (3). After 7 days the spleen is removed and the colonies counted. Knowing the number of bone-marrow cells injected, it is possible to calculate the number of stem cells which were injected. Histological examination of the colonies will show whether they were derived from the most primitive stem cells, which are capable of giving rise to all blood cell types.

cell, itself derived from the CFU-S which has undergone a stage of commitment to a particular cell lineage. Both types are capable of self-renewal. The number of multi-lineage colonies formed in the spleen of an irradiated mouse can be used to estimate the number of haemopoietic stem cells within the bone marrow as a linear relationship exists between the two.

In vitro *assay for CFU.* It has for some years been possible to grow colonies derived from haemopoietic stem cells *in vitro* (Fig. 6.4). Individual bone-marrow stem cells will grow and form colonies in semi-solid media such as 'sloppy' agar (0.3%–0.5% in tissue culture medium). Such agar does not set solid but still allows individual colonies to remain discrete as long as the right numbers of cells are used in the first place. Individual colonies can be picked up from the agar by micro-manipulation and examined histologically or re-cloned in order to examine their capacity for self-renewal. The *in vitro* colony-forming assay has revolutionized the study of haemopoiesis, particularly in humans where the spleen colony assay is obviously inappropriate. Moreover, this assay has allowed the identification of a number of 'colony-stimulating factors' (CSF) (Nicola and Vadas, 1984), in the conditioned media of several different types of cells, which promote the growth in these cultures of different lineages of blood cells. Whereas some CSFs could promote the production of one, or at most two cell types, other CSFs can support the growth of several lineages. Of the latter, IL-3 has the broadest action and for this reason is sometimes known as multi-CSF. Table 6.3 lists the major CSFs of man and the mouse, including IL-3, as well as the cellular source of these factors. In the agar colony assay, different types of colony are produced depending on the CSF present and the relative concentrations. For example, G-CSF gives rise, in mice, to colonies containing only granulocytes (although in humans it may produce mixed colonies), whereas GM-CSF at high concentration favours neutrophil formation and at low concentration favours monocytes/macrophages. Each colony originates from a stem cell or CFU although the most primitive stem cells giving rise ultimately to erythrocytes are called burst-forming units (BFU-E). Both GM-CSF and multi-CSF (IL-3) can be regarded as lymphokines since both are the products of activated T-lymphocytes, but, whereas GM-CSF can be produced by other sources such as fibroblasts, T-lymphocytes remain the sole source of IL-3.

Table 6.3 Major colony stimulating factors (CSF) of man and mouse

CSF	Cells promoted
G-CSF	Neutrophilic PMNs
GM-CSF	Granulocytes and macrophages
M-CSF	Macrophages
Multi-CSF (IL-3)	Erythrocytes, megakaryocytes, neutrophils, macrophages and mast cells
Erythropoietin	Erythrocytes

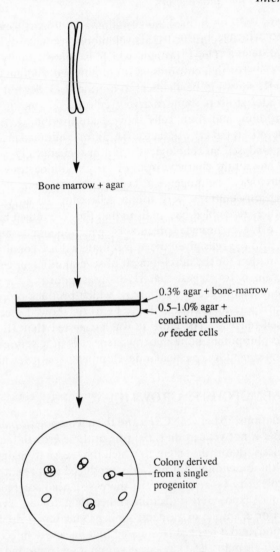

Fig. 6.4 Growth of stem cells in 'soft' agar cultures. Bone marrow is mixed with 0.3% agar in tissue culture medium at temperatures just above the setting point. The cells are layered above agar containing feeder cells or conditioned medium. Each stem cell gives rise to a colony which can be removed by micro-manipulation, and the cells examined histologically.

IL-3 AND BONE MARROW CULTURES

Several years before the association between IL-3 and the induction of 20αSDH was discovered, a growth factor present in the conditioned medium from WEHI-3B, a murine leukaemic cell line, was being used to support the long-term growth of bone marrow cultures in medium containing hydrocortisone (Greenberger *et al.*, 1983). WEHI-3B is classified as a myelomonocytic leukaemia, although the cells also express the Thy-1 protein which is more usually found on T-lymphocytes. The growth factor present in conditioned medium from these cells was subsequently shown to be identical to murine IL-3. Several permanent cell lines were produced from bone marrow cultures grown in the WEHI-3B conditioned medium and these cells showed an absolute dependence on the presence of the WEHI-3B growth factor (IL-3) for continued growth. When the cell lines were analysed morphologically and histochemically, some of the cell lines obtained had all the characteristics of early granulocytes while other lines showed morphological heterogeneity, even after they were cloned. Amongst these heterogeneous cultures were found cells with the enzymic features of neutrophils, others resembled basophils in that they contained histamine, while others were early erythrocyte precursors which could complete terminal differentiation into red cells given the appropriate culture conditions. The most plausible explanation for the development of several different cell types from a single cloned cells is to suggest that IL-3 was supporting the growth of the pluripotent stem cells in the bone marrow which produce progeny which are uncommitted to a particular lineage. These stem cells showed a seemingly infinite capacity for self-renewal. Therefore it was suggested that IL-3 acts on the progeny of the pluripotent bone marrow stem cells at a very early stage, and before any commitment to a particular developmental pathway has taken place.

ROLE OF HAEMOPOIETIC GROWTH FACTORS

The possible relationship between CSFs and the haemopoietic pathway is shown in Fig. 6.5. What is not yet certain is the role of these growth factors in steady-state haemopoiesis, that is the extent to which they serve to maintain blood cell levels in a healthy individual. Since IL-3 is produced as a result of an immune response, its role may be related to the increased need for blood cells in an individual who is exposed to infection rather than to the 'everyday' blood requirements. For example, extra neutrophil production is needed to combat bacterial infection, and it has been estimated that, in severe infection, a ten-fold increase in blood granulocytes may occur within a few days and may represent the production of approximately 2×10^{11} cells. In addition, extra macrophages may be required both for antigen processing and for 'mopping up' antigen following stimulation by other lymphokines such as IFN-γ. Thus, a stimulated T-cell produces proteins which promote the production of more phagocytic cells as they are required in an immune response. The greater energy demands of an active immune response may require increased oxygen transport and hence larger numbers of red cells in the blood. Finally, the production of extra mast cells (discussed below) is particularly important in combatting parasitic infestation. IL-3 is not the only lymphokine which acts as a mast cells growth factor (MCGF) since IL-4 also promotes the growth and differentiation of these cells, in addition to synergizing with IL-3 (Hamaguchi *et al.*, 1987).

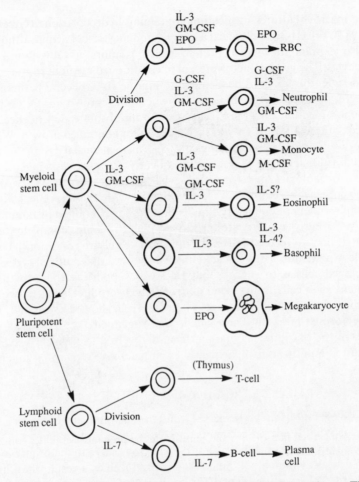

Fig. 6.5 Colony stimulating factors (CSF) and the haemopoietic pathway. The haemopoietic pathway is influenced by a number of growth factors produced by several cell types. The stages at which these growth factors possibly exert their influence is shown. (EPO = erythropoietin.)

INTERLEUKIN-3 AND MAST CELLS

Mast cells are widely distributed in the body and are found in large numbers in the skin, and linings of the respiratory and gastrointestinal tracts. These cells can be easily recognized by their characteristic morphology (Fig. 6.6) which most closely resembles that of the blood basophil. Both have prominent cytoplasmic granules containing pharmacologically active compounds such as histamine and heparin and both express membrane receptors for the Fc region of IgE (FcεR). The many similarities between mast cells and basophils has led to the proposal that blood basophils do in fact give rise to the mast cells in the solid tissues.

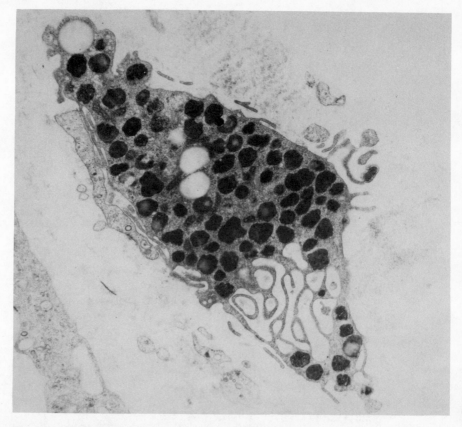

Fig. 6.6 A mast cell in a rheumatoid joint. Note the prominent granules containing pharmacological mediators. (Courtesy of Dr A. Sattar.)

Evidence for a bone marrow origin of mast cells comes from a series of elegant experiments in which strains of mice which are genetically deficient in mast cells were given a bone marrow transplant in which the cells bore a marker mutation. The recipient mice were subsequently shown to possess only mast cells bearing the same marker (Fig. 6.7) (Yung and Moore, 1985).

Role of mast cells

Mast cells are important in the development of inflammatory responses and are also implicated in the development of some allergic reactions, including hay fever and allergic asthma. In addition, the mast cell is seen to be increasingly important in the manifestation of specific immune responses to parasitic worm infestation.

Inflammation. Mast-cell mediators are important in the development of an acute inflammatory response. The release of histamine from mast cells following tissue trauma causes dilation of the blood vessels and promotes the influx of

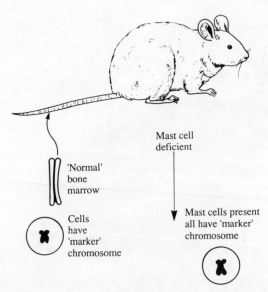

Fig. 6.7 The bone marrow origin of mast cells. Injection of 'normal' bone marrow into a mast cell-deficient mouse restores their complement of mast cells. If the injected bone-marrow cells bear a mutant chromosome marker, all the mast cells are found to have this marker.

plasma (containing antibodies and complement) and phagocytic cells into the tissues.

IgE.   Mast cells and basophils are both involved in the development of allergic reactions involving IgE. Although the development of allergic reactions in no way constitutes a 'role' for the cells, the allergic reaction probably represents an 'inappropriate' immune response, i.e. one which has another role *in vivo*. Nonetheless, a brief description of the development of such allergic reactions may provide a clue to the 'real' role of IgE *in vivo*. Allergic reactions occur when there is an inherited tendency to produce IgE rather than IgG. IgE produced in the immune response binds to the surface FcεR on mast cells and basophils (Fig. 6.8a). Further contact with the antigen (or allergen in this case) may result in the cross-linking of cell-bound IgE by antigen. If this happens, an explosive degranulation of the mast cells occurs, and the pharmacologically active factors in the mast cells are released. In addition, mast cells and basophils produce and release leukotrienes during an allergic reaction (Fig. 6.8b). A mixture of several leukotrienes constitutes the slow reacting substance of anaphylaxis (SRS-A) which causes prolonged contraction of smooth muscle such as is seen in allergic asthma. The release of all these factors locally or systemically can cause allergic reactions ranging from trivial, such as a skin rash after eating shellfish, to very serious, such as anaphylactic shock which can result in the death of a patient after exposure to an allergen (Mygind, 1986).

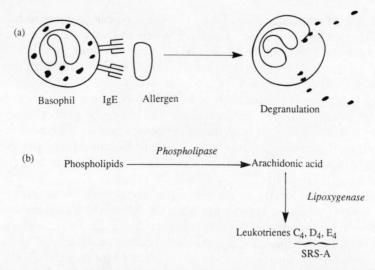

Fig. 6.8 Allergic response involving IgE and basophils/mast cells. (a) IgE, produced in response to an immunogen binds to the high-affinity FcεR on basophils or mast cells. When the IgE is at a sufficient density, the specific immunogen cross-links the IgE antibodies, triggering degranulation and release of pharmacological mediators. (b) As well as degranulation, cross-linking of IgE at the mast-cell surface activates phospholipase and triggers the production of arachidonic acid from membrane phospholipids. The membrane-associated enzyme, lipoxygenase catalyses the production of leukotrienes including leukotrienes C4, D4 and E4, which collectively make up the slow-reacting substance of anaphylaxis (SRS-A). SRS-A produces a prolonged contraction of smooth muscles and accounts for much of the respiratory distress experienced by asthmatics.

Parasites.   The allergic response mediated by IgE may represent an inappropriate manifestation of a response intended for parasites, particularly for parasitic worms. When rats are experimentally infected with nematodes, the number of mast cells in the gut mucosa increases rapidly. This increase appears to be due to immature cells in the gut being stimulated to differentiate, rather than to the entry of mature mast cells from elsewhere. The release of pharmacological mediators from mast cells may facilitate elimination of the worms. For example, both histamine and SRS-A cause contraction of the smooth muscle of the gut and this physical action may assist expulsion of the worms.

THE INVOLVEMENT OF T-LYMPHOCYTES IN MAST-CELL DEVELOPMENT

Over 25 years ago it was shown that cultures of thymus cells from outbred strains of mice frequently gave rise to large numbers of mast cells (Ginsburg and Sachs,

1963). Some 10 years later it was found that the mast-cell response to parasitic worm infection only occurred in animals which had an intact T-cell system (Ruitenberg and Elgersma, 1976). Several observations along these lines led to suggestions that mast cells are in fact derived from T-lymphocytes but this idea has not received much support. In fact, the involvement of T-lymphocytes in mast-cell development is most likely to be in the production of a growth factor which stimulates mast-cell differentiation and supports their growth. For example, when lymphocytes from helminth-infected rats are challenged *in vitro* with antigen, they release a factor into the culture medium which can stimulate· the proliferation of mast cells from cultured rat bone marrow. This factor is now established as IL-3..

When spleen cells from mice are grown for several weeks in the presence of Con-A conditioned medium, the predominant cell in these cultures strongly resembles mast cells, both morphologically, being granular, and by the expression of FcεR. This cell type was called the P or 'persisting' cell and hence the factor in Con-A supernatants which was essential for its growth was called the P cell stimulating factor (PSF) (Schrader *et al.*, 1981). The techniques of limiting dilution analysis have been applied to P cells and clones have been produced which, because they are dependent on PSF, can be used to assay the factor. These lines generally do not proliferate indefinitely even in the continued presence of PSF, and they die out after a maximum of 6 months. The development of cell lines similar to P cells is not confined to spleen cell populations and mast cells have been shown to develop from long-term cultures of bone marrow grown in the presence of media from lectin-stimulated lymphocytes. This led to the proposition that the conditioned medium contained a mast-cell growth factor (MCGF), most likely the same as PSF. Again, the continuous presence of MCGF is absolutely essential for the growth of these cells. 'P' cell lines differ from those heterogeneous self-renewing clones which can also develop in IL-3-stimulated bone marrow cultures in that they are homo-geneous, strongly resemble mucosal mast cells and have a limited life-span in culture.

CONNECTIVE TISSUES MAST CELLS (CTMC) AND MUCOSAL MAST CELLS (MMC)

In several species, including rats and mice, it is possible to distinguish two different types of mast cells based on several criteria such as their tissue location and staining characteristics (Jarrett and Haig, 1984). Mucosal mast cells (MMC) are located principally in the mucosae of the gastrointestinal and respiratory tracts whereas connective-tissue mast cells (CTMC) are found elsewhere, for example in the skin and muscular layers of the gut or around blood vessels. Infection of rats with parasitic worms results in an increase in the MMC as opposed to the CTMC. It is this increase which is dependent on the factors produced by an intact T-lymphocyte system. In addition, P cells which emerge from bone marrow and spleen cell cultures grown in the presence of IL-3 most closely resemble these MMC. A subset of mast cells equivalent to murine MMC have also been found in humans and these are present in higher numbers in the intestinal mucosae of individuals suffering from parasitic worm infections.

Molecular biology of IL-3

The biochemical analysis of lymphokines requires larger amounts of protein than are generally found in the supernatants of Con-A-activated spleen cells. Two forms of murine IL-3 have been used for studying the structure of this protein: 'native' IL-3 produced by WEHI-3B, and recombinant IL-3 using a cDNA derived from WEHI-3B IL-3-specific mRNA. The elucidation of the amino acid sequence, either by analysis of the polypeptide or by prediction from the cDNA, has enabled the entire polypeptide to be synthesized in a peptide synthesizer and this has been useful for analysing the sites which are essential for its activity.

ANALYTICAL ASPECTS

WEHI-3B conditioned medium

The murine myelomonocytic leukaemia, WEHI-3B, produces IL-3 constitutively and conditioned medium from these cells can contain up to 200 times more IL-3 than is found in the supernatants of Con-A-stimulated lymphocytes. The cells are easy to culture and can be grown at high densities in 50-litre fermenters. For these reasons, WEHI-3B was the major source of murine IL-3 prior to gene cloning. Mouse IL-3 has been purified to homogeneity from large volumes of WEHI-3B conditioned medium. The purification procedures used initially employed a variety of chromatographic procedures including ion-exchange chromatography and HPLC and yielded up to 10 μg of pure protein from 150 litres of WEHI-3B supernatant (Ihle *et al.*, 1982).

Separation of the protein by SDS–PAGE indicated that IL-3 activity resided in glycoproteins with molecular weights ranging from 28 to 32.5 kDa, with most activity occurring in the 28 kDa forms. The differences in molecular weights is entirely due to carbohydrate and the polypeptides which are obtained from these forms after treatment with neuraminidase (which removes the carbohydrate) are identical. The polypeptide obtained from WEHI-3B supernatants has 134 amino acids, six fewer than would be predicted from the corresponding cDNA. These extra six amino acids of the predicted polypeptide are found at the N-terminal end of the molecule, the remainder showing complete identity with the WEHI-3B factor.

Recombinant IL-3

The complementary DNA for murine IL-3 has been synthesized using messenger RNA isolated from WEHI-3B cells (Fung *et al.*, 1984). The cDNA has been sequenced and this has allowed the amino acid sequence of the translation product to be predicted. The cDNA codes for a protein with a molecular weight of 16 kDa, containing 166 amino acids which includes a signal sequence of 20 residues at the N-terminal end. The chromosomal gene for murine IL-3 has also been isolated and a comparison with the cDNA reveals the presence of 5 exons.

Synthetic IL-3

Knowledge of the entire amino acid sequence of IL-3 has meant that the protein can be synthesized using an automated peptide synthesizer (Clark-Lewis *et al.*, 1986). The synthesizer can be programmed to attach amino acids, in a stepwise fashion, by chemical means, to a high degree of accuracy. When the polypeptide has been synthesized, the molecule is folded by oxidizing the sulphydryl groups on cysteine molecules to yield disulphide bridges. Thus, a tertiary structure could be produced, the faithfulness to the natural molecule being analysed by comparing the peptides which are obtained from the native and synthetic molecule after limited digestion with trypsin. Complete synthesis and folding of 500 mg of IL-3 was achieved in 12 days which is a tremendous feat of protein engineering. The synthetic molecule was shown to have biological activity *in vivo*. The usefulness of this technique, though, lies not so much in producing the protein, which can after all be produced more rapidly in cell-free protein synthesizing systems, but in analysing the regions of the molecule which are essential for its activity. For example, different lengths of the peptide can be produced and tested in biological systems and peptide analogues with single or multiple amino acid substitutions can readily be synthesized. The entire IL-3 molecule was first synthesized and analysed in this way in 1986 and the results from these very elegant experiments can be summarized as follows:

- The synthetic 140 amino acid molecule was found to contain all the activities of the natural molecule
- The first six amino acids were not essential to the activity of the molecule
- A synthetic peptide containing only amino acids 1–79 could stimulate the growth of IL-3 dependent cell lines, although the activity of this fragment is very much lower than the intact molecule
- The cysteine residue at position 17 is essential to the biological activity of the molecule, possible because it is involved in a disulphide link which stabilizes the tertiary structure of the polypeptide
- Residues 7–16 are needed for maximal activity although synthetic molecules containing 17–140 do have approximately one-third of the activity of the whole molecule

Native murine IL-3 is heavily glycosylated, and approximately 36% of the weight of the molecule is due to carbohydrate which is attached at four sites on the peptide. The carbohydrate is not essential for biological activity as can be demonstrated with rIL-3 and synthetic IL-3.

MECHANISM OF ACTION OF IL-3

IL-3 interacts with cells via a receptor present on the target cell and IL-3-dependent cell lines have been shown to remove or 'absorb' IL-3 activity from WEHI-3B supernatants. The binding affinity (K_d), which has been measured by following the binding of radiolabelled IL-3 to these cell lines has been estimated to be between K_d values of 5×10^{-12} M and 5×10^{-11} M which are well within the range expected for lymphokine–receptor interactions (Crapper *et al.*, 1985). IL-3 dependent cell lines have approximately 1000 receptors per cell and polyclonal antisera prepared against IL-3 receptors can mimic the effects of IL-3 in stimulating the proliferation of these cells. Little is known about the nature of the biochemical events which take place after receptor–ligand interaction beyond the fact that the molecule is internalized and the receptors are recycled. An increase in the level of cAMP and a redistribution of membrane protein kinase-C are two subsequent events which have been measured (Whitton and Dexter, 1983; Farrar *et al.*, 1985).

HUMAN INTERLEUKIN-3

The discovery in mice of a factor which could promote the growth of several lineages of blood cells and which was produced as a result of a specific immune response was very exciting. The fact that IL-3 was routinely present in activated T-cell supernatants implied that this was a normal feature of the immune response, not only towards bacteria and viruses, but also towards parasitic worms.

The development of the agar colony assay has meant that human haemopoietic cells are now as amenable to study as are those of rodents and has shown that humans also produce CSFs analogous to the murine forms. While IL-3 is readily detectable in mice it is present only at very low levels in activated human T-lymphocyte-conditioned medium which on the other hand is a rich source of GM-CSF. Indeed, until recently, many people doubted the existence of human IL-3. Primate IL-3 was recently discovered in supernatants obtained from the gibbon T-cell line MLA 144 (which is also a constitutive producer of IL-2). MLA 144 was shown to produce GM-CSF as well as a factor which supports the growth of multi-lineage colonies when tested *in vitro* on human bone marrow cells. The cDNA encoding this activity was found to have homology with cDNA encoding murine IL-3, indicating that this factor was indeed gibbon IL-3. Since it could stimulate human bone marrow cells, it was assumed that there would be significant homology also with a putative human IL-3. The gibbon cDNA was

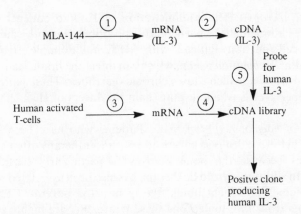

Fig. 6.9 Cloning of human IL-3. MLA-144 is a gibbon lymphoblastoid line which produces IL-3. This gibbon IL-3 was found to have a high degree of homology with mouse IL-3. mRNA isolated from MLA-144 (1) was used to produce a cDNA (2). Messenger RNA from activated human T-lymphocytes (3) was used to prepare a cDNA library in *E. coli* (4) and the clones producing human IL-3 were identified by probing with the gibbon cDNA (5).

used, successfully, to probe for human IL-3 which has subsequently been cloned (Fig. 6.9) (Yang *et al.*, 1986). Human and gibbon IL-3 are almost identical in terms of their amino acid sequence with only 11 differences between them. Structural similarities are therefore also seen between human and murine IL-3 genes in terms of exon and intron structure and some sequence homology exists over the entire molecule. The genes for human IL-3 and GM-CSF lie close together on the long arm of chromosome 5, a region which also contains the genes for several other growth factors including M-CSF and its receptor. This region has been recently examined in patients with a variety of haematological disorders including anaemia and leukaemia. Although the numbers of patients in the study were small, there did seem to be an association between the loss of IL-3 due to deletion of a small segment of chromosome 5 and haematological disease (LeBeau *et al.*, 1987).

Human IL-3 has not yet been purified from activated T-lymphocytes but the recombinant molecule is similar to murine in size, the mature peptide being 14–15 kDa in size. When the cDNA is expressed in mammalian cells, the protein is heavily glycosylated, and has a molecular weight of 30 kDa. Human IL-3, like the murine form, has a disulphide bridge which is essential for its activity.

Both gibbon and human IL-3 have multi-CSF activity and support the growth of bone marrow stem cell-derived colonies containing multiple lineages of cells.

Human IL-3 and disease

Several possibilities for the therapeutic use of human IL-3 have already been suggested and these are discussed overleaf.

Anti-parasite therapy.   The administration of IL-3 to patients with chronic parasitic infestation might be particularly appropriate for those individuals with impaired T-cell function. Patients with AIDS, for example, frequently suffer infections with *Toxoplasma gondii*, which can infect the brain, leading to seizure, and *Cryptosporidium*, which causes chronic diarrhoea. These patients have low levels of helper T-cells which are the main producers of IL-3.

Restoration of haemopoietic function.   Patients who have been irradiated or treated with cytotoxic drugs as part of an anticancer therapy often have impaired haemopoiesis because the bone marrow is particularly sensitive to these treatments. In addition, cytotoxic therapy has also been associated with deletions of chromosome 5, which holds the genes for several CSFs including IL-3. Patients who have undergone these treatments are highly susceptible to infection and may benefit from treatment with recombinant CSF. Patients whose bone marrow has been suppressed by therapeutic treatment also have low platelet levels which result in poor blood clotting. Since IL-3 supports the development of megakaryocytes *in vitro* (unlike GM-CSF) it may have therapeutic benefit in this respect also.

Patients who have been through severe trauma, such as extensive burns, and patients with some diseases, especially AIDS, may have very low neutrophil levels, a condition known as neutropenia. Again, these patients are also highly susceptible to infections, and may benefit from exogenous IL-3 (or GM-CSF).

Myelodysplasia is a stem-cell disorder which results in ineffective haemopoiesis and is associated with severe neutropenia. Patients with myelodysplasia are prone to infection and may benefit from treatment with IL-3 (Clark and Kamen, 1987; Cosman, 1988).

In addition to its possible use in treating disease, IL-3 may itself be associated with some disease. For example, in patients suffering from chronic allergic reactions such as coeliac disease, characterized by severe local reactions to gluten or wheat protein, the production of IL-3 by activated T-cells will increase the number of local mast cells and may exacerbate the disease. In these patients it may be possible to alleviate some symptoms by blocking the effect of IL-3, perhaps by administration of a specific monoclonal antibody.

Another possibility is that IL-3 might itself be associated with malignant change. IL-3 is a growth factor which, in health, affects only those cells with receptors for it. As such, a situation could be envisaged in which the gene for IL-3 production, which is normally induced during an immune response, becomes 'switched on' inappropriately, in a cell which also has receptors for it. The murine cell line WEHI-3B has been found to have a retrovirus inserted close to the gene for IL-3 and this may account for the constitutive production of IL-3 in these cells (Ymer *et al.*, 1985). Clonal analysis of IL-3-dependent lines has revealed that only cells which produce IL-3, even if in very low quantities, are capable of growing in its absence. Moreover, these cloned cells are capable of causing leukaemias if they are injected into animals from the same inbred strain (syngeneic). The gene for murine IL-3 has been inserted into IL-3 dependent cell lines derived from bone marrow, using a retroviral expression vector. Such cells have the synthesis of IL-3 permanently 'switched on' with the consequence that not only are they independent of exogenous IL-3 but they also cause leukaemia when injected into syngeneic animals. Similar results have been obtained with GM-CSF. As GM-CSF can also be regarded as a lymphokine, since it is found in activated T-cell supernatants, a brief discussion of this molecule is included in this chapter for completeness.

GM-CSF

GM-CSF is a growth factor which stimulates the production of neutrophils, eosinophils and cells of the monocyte/macrophage series. GM-CSF has been isolated from several sources including endothelial cells and fibroblasts and the conditioned media from cultures of placentas. The supernatants of activated T-lymphocytes have also been shown to contain significant activity attributable to GM-CSF and thus, like IL-3, it may be involved in the immune response-induced increases in blood cell numbers. Human GM-CSF has been produced by recombinant DNA technology using a cDNA library constructed from mRNA obtained from a human T-cell line (HUT-102) (Clark and Kamen, 1987; Cosman, 1988). Like IL-3, GM-CSF is a protein of 14–15 kDa, with extensive glycosylation (yielding 30 kDa). In addition to influencing the production of granulocytes and macrophages, GM-CSF synergizes with erythropoietin to support the production of erythrocytes and megakaryocytes and it also acts on mature granulocytes and macrophages to increase their phagocytic and bactericidal activity.

Recombinant human GM-CSF cloned in yeast cells has been used in treating human disease (Vadhan-Raj *et al.*, 1987; Cosman, 1988). Testing in primates showed that infusion of GM-CSF into monkeys resulted in a five-fold increase in total white-cell counts within 48 h. These elevated white-cell counts remained high so long as treatment continued, but rapidly returned to normal when treatment was stopped. GM-CSF has also been used to treat neutropenia in patients with AIDS and has been administered to patients with myelodysplasia. Treatment produced an increase in granulocyte levels in all patients and in some the numbers were increased several hundred times above the base level. GM-CSF also stimulates the production of monocytes and eosinophils but at higher doses than are required for the production of granulocytes. The treatment has very few toxic side effects compared with IL-2, the most common being bone pain, fever, chills, headache, loss of appetite and nausea. The bone pain is probably related to the number of stimulated cells in the bone marrow.

The therapeutic use of GM-CSF is still in its infancy and a great deal more is to be expected in the next few years. The general lack of toxicity of this growth factor and its effectiveness in increasing granulocyte numbers must instil optimism about the use of IL-3, which, like human GM-CSF, has multi-lineage activity. One significant problem with GM-CSF is the fact that it has been shown to promote the growth of myeloid leukaemic cells *in vitro*. Thus, attempts to restore white-cell counts in patients with myeloid leukaemia who have been brought into remission by cytotoxic therapy must be viewed with extreme caution. An alternative viewpoint is rather more optimistic since GM-CSF has also been shown to induce differentiation of myeloid leukaemic cells in culture. Since increased differentiation is related to a loss of the capacity to divide, it may prove that the administration of GM-CSF could turn out to have a therapeutic effect in patients with leukaemia. These uncertainties will only be resolved by extensive clinical trials which have already begun in this country and abroad. The results are awaited with intense interest both by clinicians and the commercial producers of IL-3 and GM-CSF.

Summary

The lymphokine, interleukin-3 (IL-3), promotes the production and differentiation of multiple blood cell types including granulocytes, monocytes, erythrocytes and megakaryocytes, and stimulates the production of mucosal mast cells from bone-marrow stem cells. Its effects on lymphocytes may be limited to stimulation of an early differentiation stage that is associated with the acquisition of the enzyme 20αSDH, although this enzyme is no longer considered an exclusive marker of T-lymphocytes. Human IL-3 has recently been cloned and shares some similarities with human GM-CSF, which is also detectable in the supernatants of activated T-cells. The similarities between the two molecules extend to some shared activities, to amino acid sequence homology and to the location of their respective genes which are closely linked on chromosome 5. Both lymphokines may prove to be of therapeutic use in a variety of conditions characterized by low blood cell counts, particularly of granulocytes. GM-CSF has already been tested in humans with spectacular effects on neutrophil levels and with minimal toxicity. More extensive trials of IL-3 will no doubt follow greater availability of the recombinant molecule.

References

Clark, S. C. and Kamen, R. (1987). 'The human haemopoietic colony-stimulating factors', *Science* **236**, p. 1229.
Clark-Lewis, I., Aebersold, R., Ziltener, H. *et al.* (1986). 'Automated chemical synthesis of a protein growth factor for haemopoietic cells, interleukin-3'. *Science* **231**, p. 134.
Cosman, D. (1988). 'Colony-stimulating factors *in vivo* and *in vitro*', *Immunol. Today* **9**, p. 97.
Crapper, R. M., Clark-Lewis, I. and Schrader, J. W. (1985). 'Analysis of the binding of a

haemopoietic growth factor, P-cell stimulating factor, to a cell surface receptor using quantitative absorption of bioactivity', *Exp. Haematol.* **13**, p. 941.

Farrar, W. L., Thomas, T. P. and Anderson, W. B. (1985). 'Altered cytosol enzyme redistribution on interleukin-3 activation of protein kinase-C', *Nature (London)* **315**, p. 235.

Fung, M. C., Hapel, A. J., Ymer, S., Cohen, D. R. *et al.* (1984). 'Molecular cloning of cDNA for murine interleukin-3'. *Nature (London)* **307**, p. 233.

Garland, J. M. and Dexter, T. M. (1982). '20-Alpha-hydroxysteroid dehydrogenase expression in haemopoietic cell culture and its relationship to interleukin-3', *Eur. J. Immunol.* **12**, p. 998.

Ginsburg, H. and Sachs, L. (1963). 'Formation of pure suspensions of mast cells in tissue culture by differentiation of lymphoid cells from mouse thymus', *J. Natl Acad. Sci.* **31**, p. 1.

Greenberger, J. S., Sakakeeny, M. A., Humphries, R. K. *et al.* (1983). 'Demonstration of permanent factor-dependent multipotential (erythroid/neutrophil/basophil) haematopoietic progenitor cell lines', *Proc. Natl Acad. Sci. (USA)* **80**, p. 2931.

Hamaguchi, Y., Hanakura, Y., Fujita, J. *et al.* (1987). Interleukin-4 as an essential factor for *in vitro* clonal growth of murine connective tissue-type mast cells. *J. Exp. Med.* **165**, p. 268.

Hapel, A. J., Osborne, J. M., Fung, M. C. *et al.* (1985). 'Expression of 20-alpha-hydroxysteroid dehydrogenase in mouse macrophages, haemopoietic cells and cell lines and its induction by colony-stimulating factors', *J. Immunol.* **134**, p. 2492.

Ihle, J. N. (1985). 'Biochemical and biological properties of interleukin-3: a lymphokine mediating the differentiation of a lineage of cells that includes prothymocytes and mastlike cells' in *Contemporary Topics in Molecular Immunology*, Vol. 10, *The Interleukins*, Eds Gillis, S. and Inman, F. P. London, Plenum Press.

Ihle, J. N., Pepersack, L. and Rebar, L. (1981). 'Regulation of T cell differentiation: *in vitro* induction of 20-alpha-hydroxysteroid dehydrogenase in splenic lymphocytes from athymic mice by a unique lymphokine', *J. Immunol.* **126**, p. 2184.

Ihle, J. N., Keller, J., Henderson, L. *et al.* (1982). 'Procedure for the purification of IL-3 to homogeneity', *J. Immunol.* **129**, p. 2431.

Ihle, J. N., Keller, J. Oroszlan, S. *et al.* (1983). 'Biological properties of homogeneous interleukin-3. I. Demonstration of Wehi-3 growth factor activity, mast cell growth factor activity, P cell stimulating factor activity, colony stimulating factor activity and histamine-producing cell-stimulating activity', *J. Immunol.* **131**, p. 282.

Jarrett, E. E. E. and Haig, D. M. (1984). 'Mucosal mast cells *in vivo* and *in vitro*', *Immunol. Today* **5**, p. 115.

LeBeau, M. M., Epstein, N. D., O'Brien, S. J. *et al.* (1987). 'The interleukin-3 gene is located on human chromosome 5 and is deleted in myeloid leukaemias with a deletion of 5q', *Proc. Natl. Acad. Sci. (USA)* **84**, p. 5913.

Mosmann, T. R. and Coffman, R. L. (1987). 'Two types of mouse helper T cell clone – implications for immune regulation', *Immunol. Today* **8**, p. 223.

Mygind, N. (1986). *Essential Allergy*. Oxford, Blackwell Scientific Publications.

Nicola, N. A. and Vadas, M. (1984). 'Hemopoietic colony stimulating factors', *Immunol. Today* **5**, p. 76.

Ruitenberg, E. J. and Elgersma, A. (1976). 'Absence of intestinal mast cell response in congenitally athymic mice during *Trichinella spiralis* infection', *Nature (London)* **264**, p. 258.

Schrader, W., Lewis, S. J., Clark-Lewis, I. and Culvenor, J. G. (1981). 'The persisting (P) cell: histamine content, regulation by a T cell-derived factor, origin from a bone marrow precursor, and relationship to mast cells', *Proc. Natl Acad. Sci. (USA)* **78**, p. 323.

Vadhan-Raj, S. *et al.* (1987). 'Effects of rHu GM-CSF in patients with myelodysplastic syndromes', *New Engl. J. Med.* **317**, p. 1545.

Weiss, L. (1984). *The Blood Cells and Hematopoietic Tissues*, Amsterdam, Elsevier.

Whitton, A. D. and Dexter, T. M. (1983). 'Effects of haemopoietic growth factor on intracellular ATP levels', *Nature (London)* **303**, p. 629.

Yang, Y. C. Ciarletta, A. B., Temple, P. A. *et al.* (1986). 'Human IL-3 (multi-CSF): identification by expression cloning of a novel haemopoietic growth factor related to murine IL-3', *Cell* **47**, p. 3.

Ymer, S., Tucker, W. Q. J., Sanderson, C. J. *et al.* (1985). 'Constitutive synthesis of interleukin-3 by the myelomonocytic leukaemia WEHI-3B is due to a retroviral insertion near the gene', *Nature (London)* **317**, p. 255.

Yung, Y-P. and Moore, M. A. S. (1985). 'Mast-cell growth factor: its role in mast-cell differentiation, proliferation and maturation' in *Contemporary Topics in Molecular Immunology*, Vol. 10, *The Interleukins*, Eds Gillis, S. and Inman, F. P. London, Plenum Press.

7

B-cell Growth and Differentiation Factors. Interleukins 4, 5 and 7

Introduction

The growth and differentiation of B-lymphocytes, from stem cell to plasma cell, is controlled throughout the life of the cell by a network of lymphokines and interleukins, some of which have only been characterized very recently. A list of factors which are known to control B-cell development and activation would include IL-1, IL-2, IL-4, IL-5, IL-6, IL-7, IFN-γ and TNF. In addition, there are several other less well-defined activities which will no doubt be 'cloned' and characterized in the very near future. The role of IL-1, IL-2, TNF and IFN-γ in humoral immunity is discussed in the relevant chapters devoted to each of these molecules and so will not be detailed here. Neither is it the intention to discuss those factors which have not yet been characterized: no doubt several of these will be available as recombinant molecules in the near future.

Interleukins 4, 5 and 6 are all involved in the immunological 'pathway' which starts with an antigen-specific B-lymphocyte and ends with a clone of plasma cells secreting specific antibodies. In particular, they form part of the mechanism by which 'help' is delivered by T-lymphocytes in the response to antigens which are said to be 'T-dependent'. In doing so, they may also influence the class, or isotype, of antibody which is produced. Interleukin-7 is a lymphopoietin, that is, a haemopoietic growth factor for lymphocytes and is the most recently characterized of all the interleukins. As might be expected, IL-4, 5 and 6 can influence the activity of a variety of cells apart from B-lymphocytes and even IL-7 which is, so far as is known, quite restricted in its activities, can support the proliferation of early thymocytes as well as B-lymphocytes. IL-4 and IL-5 are growth factors for mast cells and eosinophils, respectively, and as such are extremely important in the immune response towards parasites. IL-6 has so many activities in addition to its stimulation of B-cells that Chapter 8 is entirely devoted to this molecule.

Development of B-lymphocytes

In mammals, B-lymphocytes originate in, and are processed by, the fetal liver. In adult life, this function is taken over by the bone marrow which is the main centre for haemopoiesis. The pluripotent stem cells give rise, by division, to cells initially capable of developing into any type of blood cell. At a later stage there is a progressive commitment to B-cell morphology and function. This process is influenced by both internal and external factors (with respect to the bone marrow). Internal influences include both the localized micro-environments created by bone-marrow stromal cells and local concentrations of growth factors. External influences can include an active infection, which stimulates an immune response and gives rise to lymphokines or monokines which influence the proliferation of B-cell precursors.

The development of B-cells from primitive stem cells can be followed to some extent by looking at the presence of immunoglobulin on, or in, the cells (Fig. 7.1). The earliest recognizable B-cell expresses membrane IgM molecules but prior to this, a pre-B cell has been recognized and is characterized by the presence of cytoplasmic μ-chains which are the heavy chains for IgM (Roitt, 1988). The pre-B cell develops from a pre-pre-B (or pro-B) with neither surface nor cytoplasmic heavy chains or immunoglobulin. Interleukin-7 is known to stimulate the proliferation of both pro- and pre-B lymphocytes (Henney, 1989).

As B-cells mature in the bone marrow, they may begin to express other immunoglobulin isotypes either alone or concomitantly with IgM and/or IgD. Whatever the combination of isotypes expressed within a membrane, the epitope specificity of the different isotypes expressed is always identical and this is because the same variable (V)-region genes (which contribute to the antibody-combining site) for heavy (H) and light (L) chains can be combined with different constant region genes (which in heavy chains specifies the immunoglobulin isotype). The epitope specificity of immunoglobulin within a particular B-cell is determined during ontogeny following a series of rearrangements within the DNA coding for the heavy and light chains of the immunoglobulin.

Rearrangements in immunoglobulin genes

The ability of vertebrates to produce specific antibodies to every possible epitope is truly astonishing. There seems to be no limit to the number of different antibody molecules which can be produced even against molecules to which the animal would not naturally be exposed. At the same time all antibodies mediate destruction of immunogens through a limited number of pathways such as lysis via complement activation, or stimulation of uptake by phagocytic cells. The uniqueness of an antibody molecule is determined by the variable regions of the light and heavy chains, while the amino acid sequence in the constant regions of the heavy chains (Fc) determines the biological properties of the molecule, such as its ability to activate complement, as well as determining the antibody class.

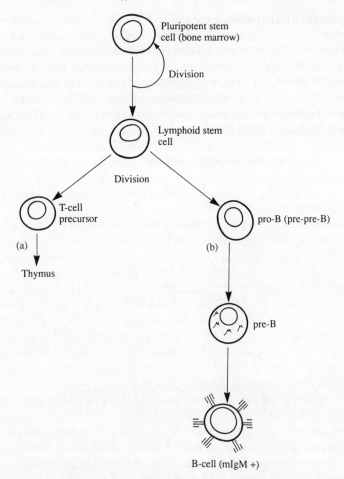

Fig. 7.1 Development of B-cells from primitive stem cells. The pluripotent stem cell (in the fetal liver and, later, in the adult bone marrow), gives rise to the lymphoid stem cell. The progeny of the lymphoid stem cell gives rise (a) to the precursors of the T-cells which are processed in the thymus and (b) to the precursors of the B-lymphocytes, the pro-B (or pre-pre-B) cell. Division of the pro-B-cell and subsequent differentiation of the progeny produces the pre-B-cell, which is recognizable by the presence of immunoglobulin μ chains in the cytoplasm. The most primitive B-cell is derived from the pre-B and expresses membrane IgM molecules.

The great diversity in antibody molecules, whereby millions of different antibody molecules can be produced from relatively small amounts of DNA is brought about by having many V genes, any of which can be joined to a particular constant region (C) gene by one of several forms of diversity (D) and joining (J) genes. Polypeptide chains can be produced from genes, which in the germ-line are not continuous, by slicing out the intervening DNA and joining the cut-ends (Fig. 7.2). In addition, cutting and splicing of mRNA transcripts may also be employed. Rearrangement of RNA would have the same end result but would not necessitate permanent changes in the DNA itself. The production of specific antibodies appears to utilize both DNA and RNA rearrangements. For simplicity, the process of gene rearrangement will only be discussed in the heavy chain since it is this chain which determines the class of antibody which is expressed. However, gene rearrangements do occur in the genes which specify both the κ- and the λ-light chains.

(a) *Splicing and joining of DNA*

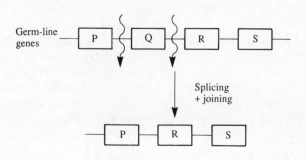

(b) *Splicing of mRNA transcript*

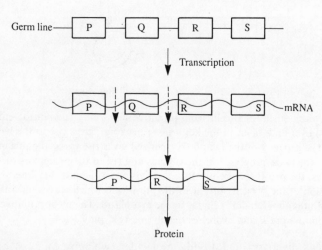

Fig. 7.2 Production of a polypeptide chain from discontinuous genes. A protein can be the product of two or more genes, even if these genes are discontinuous in the germ-line DNA. This can be brought about by a permanent splicing of the DNA in an individual cell (a), cutting out the intermediate sequences and rejoining the remaining DNA. Alternatively, splicing and rejoining of the RNA transcript can have the same effect without a permanent deletion of DNA (b).

PRODUCTION OF IMMUNOGLOBULIN HEAVY CHAINS

The genes for heavy chains are found, in man, on chromosome 14. This chromosome has several hundred V-region genes each coding for a specific amino acid sequence. The V-region genes are separated from the D genes and several J genes by intervening DNA sequences (Fig. 7.3a). Further downstream there is a stack of genes each specifying the constant regions for one of the heavy chain isotypes or subclasses. During ontogeny, deletion and rejoining of DNA segments brings together a J gene and a D gene and the JD combination next to one of the V-region genes. In this process, the intervening DNA is deleted. Considerable diversity can be achieved at this stage owing to the different possible combinations of VD and J genes and the positions at which they are joined.

Transcripts (mRNA) from this successful VDJ arrangement can be spliced to a heavy-chain transcript and translated to yield a heavy chain of a particular isotype. The transcripts of the same V, D and J genes can therefore be joined to different heavy-chain gene transcripts to produce immunoglobulins with the same specificity but different isotypes, following combination with light chains which have undergone similar gene rearrangements. When the light and the

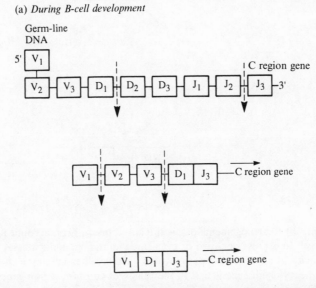

(a) *During B-cell development*

Fig. 7.3 Rearrangements in heavy chain genes. (a) Permanent rearrangements of DNA occur in B-cell development, and account for the epitope specificity of the mature B-cell, though not the class of immunoglobulin which will be produced. For simplicity only three V, D and J genes are shown. The first rearrangement brings together one D and one J gene and then the DJ complex is rearranged next to one of several hundred V genes. A transcript of the VDJ region would provide the heavy chain 'contribution' to the Fab region of the antibody.

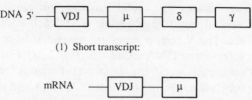

(b) *mRNA arrangements*

(1) Short transcript:

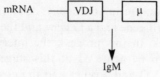

(2) Longer transcript:

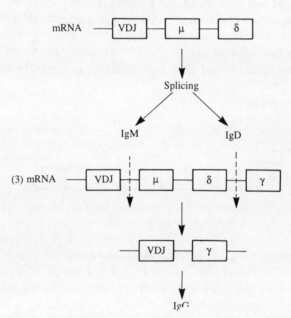

Fig. 7.3 *cont.* (b) Rearrangements of the mRNA transcript can account for the ability of a single cell to express one, two or even three immunoglobulin classes all with the same specificity. A short transcript (1) would yield a cell expressing μ chains (IgM) since the μ heavy chain gene is first in the 'stack' of constant region genes. A longer transcript (2) with splicing would allow a cell to express both IgM and IgD. In a similar fashion (3), a longer, spliced transcript would yield γ chains of IgG.

(c) *Irreversible class switch*

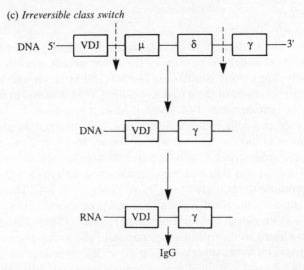

Fig. 7.3 *cont.* (c) An irreversible class switch, from a cell expressing IgM to one expressing IgG, would involve further rearrangement of the DNA.

heavy chains join to form an immunoglobulin molecule, the molecule will be expressed at the cell surface. Somatic mutation may take place in the rearranged genes which can result in the modification of the antibody combining site of expressed molecules.

The earliest recognizable B-cells express IgM and this can be attributed to the production of a short transcript (see Fig. 7.3b), the μ gene being first in the stack of heavy-chain genes, rather than to a permanent deletion of other heavy-chain constant region genes. At later stages, when the cell co-expresses IgM and another immunoglobulin, there may be rearrangement of a longer RNA transcript rather than the deletion of intervening genes. If a cell which is expressing IgM is stimulated, it will initially produce and secrete IgM molecules of identical specificity but later there may be a class switch, possibly to IgG production. Such a switch is more likely to be permanent and may be due to further gene recombination events within the DNA of the antibody-producing cell (Fig. 7.3c), although alteration of the transcript could still account for this class switch. The study of soluble factors from cloned helper T-lymphocytes has revealed that several T-cell lymphokines, including IL-4, 5 and IFN-γ can influence the class of antibody which is produced in a humoral response. At least part of the influence on the immunoglobulin isotype is exerted at the level of the class switch.

It is now possible to discuss the roles of the different lymphokines in the growth and differentiation of the B-cells and, since IL-7 exerts the earliest effects on the development of B-cells, this will be discussed first.

Interleukin-7

The pathway of differentiation which is taken by the progeny of the stem cells in the bone marrow is under the control of the haemopoietic growth factors, the best known being the colony stimulating factors (CSFs) which were discussed in Chapter 6. However, none of these CSFs, including IL-3, appears to influence the development of lymphocytes. For several years it has been known that the supporting, or stromal cells, in the bone marrow, can influence the production of B-lymphocytes in liquid cultures of bone marrow. Moreover, the conditioned media from cultured stromal cells are as effective as the cells themselves, particularly if the stromal cells had been transformed with the SV40 virus which is known to promote the activity of the 'host' genes' (Fig. 7.4). The stromal cell factor which supports the proliferation of B-cell precursors is IL-7, which until very recently was known as lymphopoietin-1 (Henney, 1989). The murine IL-7 gene has been cloned using transformed stromal cells as the source of specific mRNA. Murine cDNA was subsequently used to detect the human IL-7 gene by probing a cDNA library obtained from a human hepatoma cell line. Recombinant human IL-7 has activities similar to the murine form and promotes the proliferation of bone marrow from both species.

IL-7 stimulates the proliferation of pro- and pre-B-lymphocytes but does not appear to affect either the differentiation or the proliferation of mature B-lymphocytes.

Until recently, IL-7 was thought to act exclusively on the precursors of the B-lymphocytes but a search for mRNA coding for IL-7 has revealed its presence in mouse thymus tissue. In addition, IL-7 has been shown to stimulate the proliferation of thymocytes in the absence of mitogens such as PHA and to enhance the mitogenic effect of PHA on both thymocytes and mature T-cells.

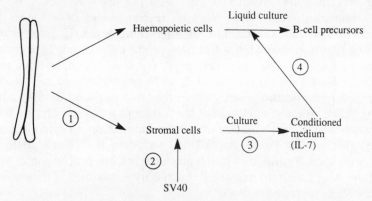

Fig. 7.4 Interleukin 7 (lymphopoietin-1). The stromal, or supporting, cells of the bone-marrow produce growth factor which influence haemopoiesis. IL-7 is produced by SV 40-transformed stromal cells in culture. The supernatants from these cells stimulate the production of B-cell precursors in liquid cultures of bone marrow.

This enhancement may be brought about by a stimulation of IL-2 production by thymus cells coupled with an increase in the expression of IL-2 receptors.

STRUCTURE OF IL-7

Complementary DNA for murine IL-7 codes for a protein of approximately 15 kDa which has two N-linked glycosylation sites. Glycosylation of the native molecule is extensive and increases the molecular weight to 25 kDa. In addition, six cysteine residues are found within the molecule, probably involved in intra-chain disulphide bonds since reduction results in the loss of activity. The murine and human forms show 60% homology at the amino acid level and this probably accounts for their biological cross-reactivity.

POTENTIAL FOR IL-7

IL-7 should be included in the list of factors with potential for stimulating the growth of depleted bone marrow. It is possible to envisage a time when such treatments involve a 'cocktail of haemopoietins' such as IL-3 and IL-7, which could be used to restore all of the cells of the bone marrow.

Interleukins 4 and 5

Interleukins 4 and 5 are the products of helper T-cells and they account for some of the means whereby T_H provides 'help' to B-cells in the production of antibody. The process of antibody production can be summarized into three components, namely, activation, proliferation and differentiation, as shown in Fig. 7.5. Most of the effects of IL-4 and IL-5 on B-cells and antibody production appear to take

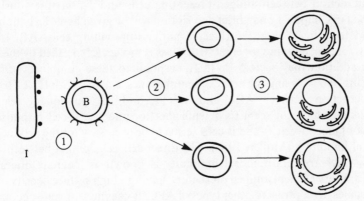

Fig. 7.5 Stages in the production of antibody. (1) Activation of the specific B-cell by epitopes on an immunogen (I). (2) Proliferation is essential for the development of specific immunity. (3) The progeny of the stimulated B-cells differentiate into plasma cells secreting specific antibody; some cells may not differentiate but remain as memory cells.

place after activation. Interleukins 4 and 5 both promote the growth and differentiation of stimulated B-cells, influencing the class and subclass of antibody which is produced during the process. In addition, IL-4 may also be involved in activation since it is known to increase the expression of MHC Class II molecules on B-cells and macrophages, and therefore may improve their capability for presenting antigen to helper T-lymphocytes (Swain *et al.*, 1988).

The nature of T-cell 'help'

The idea that T-cells provide help to B-cells in humoral immune responses was first proposed nearly 20 years ago when it became apparent that the majority of antigens fail to elicit a good antibody response in the absence of viable T-cells, for example, in neonatally thymectomized mice. Observations made in 1972, that the supernatants of activated T-cells could sometimes substitute for the cells themselves in promoting antibody production led to the extensive investigation of T-cell-replacing factors (TRFs) (Schimpl and Wecker, 1972). Interleukins 4 and 5 both account for at least some of the activity of T-cells in promoting B-cell activity. With the advent of recombinant IL-4 and IL-5 it has been possible to show that the ability to stimulate growth as well as differentiation can be vested in a single molecule, rather than in separate factors as was first thought. Moreover, the same molecule can have separate effects on a variety of cell types. Table 7.1 gives a list of 'alternative' names for these lymphokines and the different cells which are 'targets' for their activity.

Cognate interactions between B-cells and T-cells

The interaction between antigen-presenting cells and T_H has previously been described in Chapter 1 but a brief description will be given here. T_H lymphocytes respond to antigen on the surface of antigen presenting cells (APC), which present 'foreign' epitopes together with Class II molecules specified by the MHC, and in addition they secrete IL-1. T_H respond to these combined stimuli by producing and releasing the array of lymphokines, starting with IL-2. However, the interaction between APC and T-cells, and the subsequent release of lymphokines does not seem to be sufficient to influence B-cell responses and direct contact between T- and B-cells seems to be necessary for the production of humoral immunity (Moller, 1987). The direct cell–cell contact between T- and B-cells which triggers humoral immunity is known as 'cognate interaction'. B-cells are very efficient antigen presenters, having a high surface density of Class II molecules. In contrast to other types of APC, B-cells are antigen-specific which may increase their potential for presentation. It is possible that some lymphokines secreted by T_H may only work at short range or in regions of high local concentrations. Interleukins 2, 4, 5, 6 and IFN-γ are all products of T_H which are involved in B-cell activity. In mice, where two populations of T_H have been shown to have different patterns of lymphokine production (Table 7.2), IFN-γ

Table 7.1 Alternative names for IL-4 and IL-5

Interleukin designation	Name	Definition	Activity stimulated
IL-4	BCGF-I	B-cell growth factor	Co-stimulator of B-cell proliferation (with anti-IgM)
	BCGF-γ	B-cell growth factor	and preferentially stimulates IgG production
	BSF-I	B-cell stimulatory factor	Stimulates differentiation as well as growth of B-cells
	MCGF-II	Mast cell growth factor (distinct from IL-3)	Promotes growth of mucosal mast cells
	TCGF-II	T-cell growth factor (distinct from IL-2)	Promotes proliferation of T-cells
IL-5	BCGF-II	B-cell growth factor (distinct from BCGF-I)	Co-stimulator of dextran sulphate stimulated B-cells
	BCDFμ	B-cell differentiation factor	Promotes IgM production in activated B-cells
	TRF-I	T-cell replacement factor	Stimulates terminal differentiation of B-cells into plasma cells
	EDF	Eosinophil differentiation factor	Promotes production of eosinophils from bone marrow
	KHF	Killer helper factor	Promotes production of CTL from thymocytes in presence of IL-2

Table 7.2 Patterns of lymphokine production in murine T_{H1} and T_{H2} clone

Lymphokine	T_{H1}	T_{H2}
IL-2	+ +	−
IFN-γ	+ +	−
TNF-β	+ +	−
GM-CSF	+ +	+
IL-3	+ +	+ +
IL-4	−	+ +
IL-5	−	+ +
IL-6	−	+ +

Key:
  − none present   + low levels   + + high levels

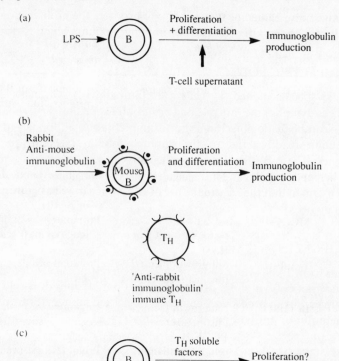

Fig. 7.6 Systems used to study T-cell 'helper' factors for B-lymphocytes. (a) LPS is a polyclonal activator of B-lymphocytes. Supernatants of T_H clones are included in the incubation mixture to assess the effect on the amount and class of antibody produced. (b) Mouse B-cells are polyclonally activated with rabbit anti-mouse immunoglobulin. Helper T-cells from mice rendered immune to rabbit immunoglobulin can be used instead of supernatants. (c) Resting B-cells have been tested with helper T-cell factors to test the effect on proliferation and antibody production.

and IL-2 are produced by T_{H1} clones and IL-4 and IL-5 by T_{H2} clones (Coffman *et al.*, 1988). Supernatants from the two different cloned helper cell populations have revealed interesting differences in the ability of these clones to provide 'help' for B-lymphocytes. The systems which have been used to study this phenomenon *in vitro* (Fig. 7.6) include the following:

LIPOPOLYSACCHARIDE (LPS) ACTIVATION OF B-CELLS

LPS is a powerful polyclonal activator of B-lymphocytes, leading to detectable immunoglobulin secretion after 4–5 days. The supernatants from the different T-cell clones have been studied for their ability to promote the proliferation of the stimulated B-cells, or to alter the class of immunoglobulin which is produced.

ANTIGEN-SPECIFIC POLYCLONAL SYSTEMS

When antigen-specific cloned T_H cells are cultured with syngeneic antigen-presenting cells, lymphokines are released *in vitro*. By choosing the right antigen, the response can be made polyclonal. For example, rabbit antibodies to mouse immunoglobulin readily bind to the immunoglobulin receptor on mouse B-lymphocytes. These B-cells can then efficiently present this rabbit immunoglobulin to helper T-cell clones generated against rabbit immunoglobulin. These systems are useful in that they avoid the use of LPS which may have direct effects on the cells involved.

RESTING B-CELLS

Supernatants from T-cells clones have been tested on resting B-cells derived from blood and a variety of lymphoid tissues. Enriched populations of B-cells can be prepared by a variety of procedures but some T-cells and monocytes are required for the generation of antibody in these systems.

Whatever system has been used to generate antibody, T_{H2} clones or the supernatants from them have invariably been shown to generate greater amounts of antibody than T_{H1} clones. This increase in immunoglobulin levels cannot be attributed to increased proliferation, since IL-2 produced by T_{H1} clones is a potent growth factor for stimulated B-cells. In addition, the pattern of immunoglobulin isotypes has been shown to be greatly influenced by the clone used.

The majority of B-cells obtained from mouse spleen express both sIgM and sIgD. When highly purified suspensions of these B-cells are stimulated with LPS, the cells proliferate and differentiate into antibody-secreting cells. The major immunoglobulin produced under these conditions is IgM but IgG_3 and IgG_{2b} are also present in significant amounts whereas others (IgG_1 and IgG_{2a}) are at low levels or may, like IgA or IgE, be undetectable. When supernatants from T_{H2} clones are added to LPS-activated B-cells, a pattern of immunoglobulin isotypes is produced which is profoundly different (Fig. 7.7). For example, there is a significant increase in the levels of IgA, IgG_1 and IgE. The greatest increase is in IgE which may be increased as much as 1000-fold. In addition to an enhancement of these isotypes, the production of the IgG_{2a} subclass is significantly decreased. One method for determining which lymphokine mediates the change in isotype patterns is to include a specific monoclonal antibody, such as anti-IL-4, in the reaction mixture. Alternatively, recombinant interleukins can be tested for their ability to substitute for the clone supernatants. Using these techniques it has been established that IL-4 stimulates the increase in IgG_1 and IgE, while IL-5 increases

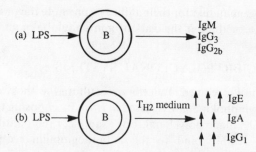

Fig. 7.7 The effect of T_{H2} supernatants on antibody class. In the presence of supernatants from T_{H2} clones, LPS-stimulated B-cells (b) produce a profoundly different pattern of immunoglobulin classes from controls (a).

the IgA content in the stimulated cultures. In addition, some synergistic effects have also been seen between IL-4 and IL-5. For example, IL-5 can enhance the IgE level in stimulated B-cell cultures when IL-4 is present in sub-optimal concentrations.

When supernatants from T_{H1} clones are used in these experiments, there is a significant increase in the level of IgG_{2a} and this is related to the presence of IFN-γ in the culture supernatants. IFN-γ has opposing effects to IL-4 on IgG_1 and IgE levels and inhibits IL-4 induction of these antibodies, particularly IgE (Coffman and Carty, 1986). Similar results have been found when whole cells have been used instead of their supernatants. Thus, it seems that the levels of IgE, IgG_1, IgA and IgG_{2a} will be controlled *in vitro* by the relative numbers of T_{H1} and T_{H2} cells at the site of B-cell stimulation. In mice, the products of T_{H1} clones are important in immunity to viruses. IgG_{2a}, for example, is involved in antiviral responses; this subclass is efficient in complement fixation and can lyse membrane-bound virions. Its level is controlled by another well-known antiviral compound, IFN-γ, and it is produced by the same cell which secretes IL-2. IL-2 is essential for the development of cytotoxic T-lymphocytes, capable of killing virus-infected cells in a specific manner. Moreover, both IL-2 and IFN-γ increase the lytic ability of NK cells which kill virus-infected cells in a non-specific manner.

The clear findings in mice, therefore, point to the presence of two helper T-cell types with quite different roles *in vivo*. T_{H2} cells stimulate the production of murine IgG_1 and IgE which in mice play a significant role in the immune response towards parasitic infections. In addition, IL-4 and IL-5 are growth factors for mast cells and eosinophils, respectively. Each of these cells is essential for the elimination of parasites.

Growth promotion and the immunoglobulin class switch

The promotion of individual immunoglobulin isotypes by proteins such as IL-4 and IL-5 could be due to one of two mechanisms:

(1) IL-4 and IL-5 may differentially influence those B-cells which are already committed to producing, say, IgE or IgA. That is, they promote those cells already expressing surface IgE or IgA, *or*

(2) IL-4 and IL-5 can increase the number of cells which express a particular isotype, by promoting the immunoglobulin class switch in these cells. This in itself may involve the stimulation of further gene rearrangements within the DNA of these cells.

In practice, it is likely that both mechanisms may play a part. For example, IL-4 is known to stimulate an isotype switch from cells expressing sIgM in favour of IgE and IgG_1-expressing cells. In contrast, the preferential stimulation of IgA by IL-5 may be due to a selective effect on cells previously expressing sIgA (i.e. cells which have already 'switched') (Snapper *et al.*, 1988).

IL-4 and FcεR

Receptors for the Fc region of IgE are found on a number of cell types. Mast cells and basophils, for example, are characterized by high-affinity receptors (FcεR-I) which are involved in the IgE-triggered release of mast cell mediators which can occur in allergic responses or in anti-parasite immunity. B-cells have low-affinity Fcε receptors (FcεR-II) which are present during B-cell differentiation but are normally lost when B-cells have switched to sIgA or IgG expression. These low-affinity receptors can therefore be regarded as a differentiation marker, and have the CD23 designation (Kikutani *et al.*, 1986). IL-4 increases the number of B-cells expressing FcεR-II and the density of these receptors on individual cells. B-cells in culture also secrete an IgE binding factor which is a cleavage product of the cell-bound receptor (soluble CD23) and which reacts with an antibody to it. The density of IgE receptors on B-cells is related to a stimulation of IgE production, possibly by an autocrine stimulation resulting from the attachment of IgE to these receptors (Hudak *et al.*, 1987; Pene *et al.*, 1988).

Human IL-4 and IL-5

Both IL-4 and IL-5 were originally discovered in mice but the genes for the equivalent molecules in humans have been identified and cloned (Yokota *et al.*, 1988). This was achieved by using gene probes based on the murine molecules, on the assumption that there would be significant homology between the human and murine forms. Although humans do produce IL-4 and IL-5, there is, as yet, little evidence for the existence of helper T-cell subsets equivalent to T_{H1} and T_{H2} subsets in humans. Many human T_H clones produce both IL-2 and IFN-γ and are thus similar to T_{H1} murine clones but others produce IL-4 and IL-5 in addition to IL-2 and IFN-γ. In one particular study of nearly 700 T_H clones, no consistent pattern of lymphokine production could be identified (Maggi *et al.*, 1988).

In spite of some amino acid sequence homology, human and murine IL-4 are species-specific. This is not the case with IL-5 and the murine molecule has activity on human cells and vice-versa. However, human IL-5 does not appear to have any growth factor activity, either on mouse or human B-cells although it does act as a differentiation factor, promoting the production of IgA. Both mouse and human IL-5 have similar effects on the differentiation of eosinophils.

Significance of IL-4 and IL-5 *in vivo*

IMMUNITY TO PARASITES

IL-4 and IL-5 undoubtedly have an important role in the host response to parasites such as helminths, nematodes and some protozoa. The involvement of these interleukins lies mainly in their effects on IgE production (IL-4); on the growth of mast cells (IL-4), and on the growth and activation of eosinophils (IL-5).

IL-4 and IgE in parasitic infections

The sera of mice which have been experimentally infected with a nematode such as *Nippostrongylus brasiliensis* have elevated levels of IgE and IgG_1 (Jarret and Miller, 1982). In addition, the spleens from infected animals secrete relatively large amounts of IL-4 in culture. Rats similarly infected have high levels of IgE binding factors in the serum which, as we have seen, are related to high levels of IgE. A monoclonal antibody to IL-4 can prevent the increase in IgE in mice if it is injected shortly after parasite infection. Paradoxically, IgG_1 levels are not affected by the administration of anti-IL-4 which may indicate that lower amounts of this lymphokine are needed for the stimulation of this subclass.

IgE and IgG_1 can both coat parasites and render them susceptible to killing by eosinophils. IgE also binds to tissue mast cells via $Fc\varepsilon R$-I (high affinity). Cross-linking of IgE molecules by antigen leads to a rapid degranulation of the mast cells with a variety of subsequent effects (Chapter 6). The pharmacological mediators in the granules and leukotrienes which are stimulated in this reaction produce a variety of effects including vasodilation, which results in inflammation, smooth muscle contraction, and the chemotactic attraction of eosinophils.

IL-4 is a mast-cell growth factor (MCGF-II)

Supernatants from mouse T_{H2} clones were shown to promote the outgrowth of mast cells from bone marrow (Nabel *et al.*, 1981; Hamaguchi *et al.*, 1987). When these supernatants were analysed, the bulk of MCGF activity was found to reside in IL-3 but an additional factor, clearly distinct from IL-3, was found both to promote mast-cell growth and to enhance the MCGF activity of IL-3. Moreover, recombinant IL-3 was never able to stimulate mast cells to the same extent as T_{H2}

supernatants. Mast cells are reservoirs of an array of pharmacological mediators which provide a defence against parasites. Since IL-4 also increases IgE, which indirectly causes degranulation of mast cells, it becomes obvious that IL-4 is very important in immunity to parasites.

IL-5 is an eosinophil differentiation factor (EDF)

Eosinophils are polymorphonuclear leukocytes which contain toxic cationic proteins in prominent secretory granules (Fig. 7.8). Compared with neutrophils they are poor phagocytes but can kill IgG-coated target both by ADCC and via complement-induced phagocytosis. Eosinophils are able to kill antibody-coated helminths (as well as other target cells) by virtue of binding to the target via Fc receptors. Following binding they release toxic cationic proteins and reactive oxygen metabolites (Butterworth, 1984; Sanderson *et al.*, 1988).

Eosinophils are produced in the bone marrow, circulate in the blood for about 12 h and then emerge in the connective tissues. The numbers in connective tissue in a healthy individual are low and similarly they make up <2% of the blood leukocytes. However, patients who suffer IgE-related allergies such as hay fever or allergic asthma, or who are infected with parasites such as *Toxocara* or *Schistosoma mansonii*, have greatly increased numbers of eosinophils, i.e. have eosinophilia. The relationship between eosinophilia and elevated IgE levels in the

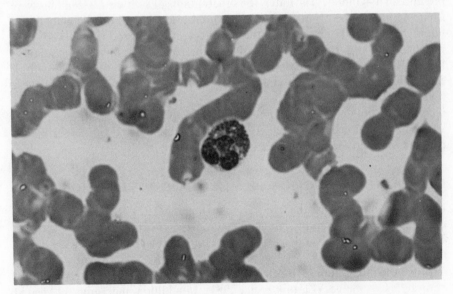

Fig. 7.8 The eosinophil. The eosinophil contains prominent cytoplasmic cationic granules which are toxic to the larvae of many parasitic worms.

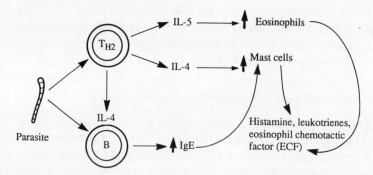

Fig. 7.9 Anti-parasite immunity. IL-4, produced by T_H during the specific immune response, promotes the production of IgE and an increase in mast-cell numbers. IgE can trigger the release of mast cell mediators, one of which is a chemotactic factor for eosinophils, which can kill parasites. The number and phagocytic activity of eosinophils is in turn stimulated by IL-5. Therefore IL-4 and IL-5 are both important in the control of parasites, although they may also be involved in the development of inappropriate hypersensitivity reactions as well.

blood has been established for a number of years although it is only in recent years that an explanation for this relationship could be proffered.

Nearly 20 years ago it was established that the experimental eosinophilia, which can be induced in rodents by injection of parasites, was dependent on the presence of T-lymphocytes. Later, the supernatants of activated spleen cells were found to induce the production of eosinophil colonies, in both semi-solid and liquid cultures of bone marrow (the latter consistently producing a very high proportion of such colonies). The active factor, called eosinophil differentiation factor (EDF) was later re-named IL-5. In addition to stimulating the growth of eosinophils, within the bone marrow, IL-5 also increases the activity of these cells. For example, eosinophils taken from patients with eosinophilia show increased cytotoxicity towards parasites *in vitro* (O'Garra *et al.*, 1986).

The interrelationship between IL-4, IL-5, eosinophilia and IgE levels in anti-parasite immunity is summarized in Fig. 7.9.

IL-4 AND THE INDUCTION OF MHC CLASS II EXPRESSION

IL-4 is known to increase the level of expression of MHC Class II antigens on B-lymphocytes as well as monocytes and macrophages (Swain *et al.*, 1988; Littman *et al.*, 1989). The effect is not so marked on human B-cells which already have a high density of Class II expression. The increase in Class II expression may improve the interaction of B-cells with T_H cells, and improve antigen presentation by macrophages (Zlotnik *et al.*, 1987). In addition, macrophages treated with IL-4 display increased tumoricidal activity although this is probably unrelated to the ability to kill tumours by non-specific means.

IL-4 IS A T-CELL GROWTH FACTOR (TCGF)

Interleukin-4 is known to support the growth of lectin-stimulated T-lymphocytes. Thus it is the second T-cell growth factor (TCGF-II) (Smith and Rennick, 1986). Similarly, supernatants from mouse T_{H2} clones with no detectable IL-2 or IL-2 specific mRNA were found to promote the growth of T-lymphocytes stimulated with PHA (Mosmann *et al.*, 1986). Extensive purification and biochemical analysis have proved that TCGF-II always co-purifies with MCGF-II and studies on the ability of rIL-4 to promote the growth of T-cells have confirmed these results.

Human IL-4 also has TCGF-II activity and supports the proliferation of activated $CD4^+$ and $CD8^+$ cells which express Class II molecules. Both human and murine IL-4 enhance the generation of specific cytotoxic T-lymphocytes (CTL) from mixed leukocyte cultures. This effect could, at least in part, be due to the TCGF activity of this lymphokine. IL-5 has also been shown to promote the induction of CTL from thymocytes in the presence of a co-stimulator and IL-2. In this case, IL-5 is thought to promote the expression of receptors for IL-2 on the thymocytes rather than the direct promotion of CTL. The activity of IL-4 as a TCGF means therefore that, at least in mice, T_{H2} clones are able to promote cell-mediated immunity in the absence of IL-2.

IL-4 AND IMMUNITY TO TUMOURS

Incubation of peripheral blood mononuclear cells with IL-2 for 48 h results in the induction of lymphokine-activated killer (LAK) cells. LAK cells are cells with cytotoxic effects on a wide range of fresh tumour cells. In mice, IL-4 has been shown to enhance LAK activity in cells which have been treated with sub-optimal concentrations of IL-2 (Mule *et al.*, 1987). Unlike NK cells, LAK are not restricted to a narrow range of cultured tumour targets. In humans, LAK therapy, involving administration of IL-2 and pre-activated autologous LAK cells to cancer patients has had some success in causing regression of established tumours. However, in humans, IL-4 does not seem to induce LAK and, in contrast, can inhibit IL-2-mediated induction of LAK. This agrees with another finding that both mouse and human IL-4 inhibit IL-2-mediated increases in NK activity. These opposing findings concerning LAK activation in the presence of IL-4 remain to be resolved.

Molecular biology of IL-4 and IL-5

The genes for murine IL-4 and IL-5 have both been cloned within the last three years. Human T-cell clones with known BCGF activity were used to prepare a DNA library which was then probed with DNA complementary to murine IL-4 and IL-5, on the assumption (fortunately correct) that there would be significant

Table 7.3   Comparison of human and mouse IL-4 and IL-5

Property	IL-4		IL-5	
	Human	*Murine*	*Human*	*Murine*
Amino acid residues (secreted)	129	120	115	113
Residues in signal sequence	24	20	19	20
Predicted size of polypeptide	15 kDa	14 kDa	14 kDa	14 kDa
Potential N-glycosylation sites	2	3	2	2
Post-glycosylation species	15, 18, 19 kDa	15, 19 kDa	20 kDa	22 kDa
Location of gene (chromosome number)	5		5	11

homology between the human and the murine forms. These techniques have enabled the human forms to be detected and cloned. Human and mouse IL-4 have distinct regions in which homology at the amino acid level approaches 50%. Human and murine IL-5 are much more similar and homology extends here to nearly 70% of the amino acid sequence.

A comparison between the molecular characteristics of human and murine IL-4 and IL-5 is shown in Table 7.3.

The genes for both murine and human IL-4 have a similar organization in that they both have 4 exons and 3 introns, as indeed do several other lymphokines such as IL-2 and IFN-γ. The gene for human IL-4 and IL-5 are located on chromosome 5 together with the genes for IL-3, GM-CSF and CSF-1 (M-CSF). Such collections of genes for haemopoietic growth factors may have important consequences for the regulation of blood cell production and complete or partial deletions in chromosome 5 are frequently observed in patients with acute non-lymphocytic leukaemia. The gene for murine IL-5 is situated on chromosome 11 on the same chromosome as the genes for IL-3 and GM-CSF. Although the location of the gene for murine IL-4 has not yet been discovered, it seems fairly likely that it will also be on chromosome 11 (Sideras *et al.*, 1988; Yokota *et al.*, 1988).

RECEPTORS

Radiolabelled IL-4 has been used to estimate the number and affinity of specific receptors on IL-4-sensitive cells. IL-4 was shown to bind to a variety of cells including haemopoietic cells. Most cell types had high-affinity receptors, the numbers ranging from several hundred to over 5000 per cell. The binding affinity (K_d) of these receptors lies in the range $2-8 \times 10^{-11}$ M. The range of receptor-positive cells is shown in Table 7.4. So far, only high-affinity receptors have been

Table 7.4   Distribution of IL-4R

- B-cells
- Mast cells
- Macrophages
- Monocytes
- Polymorphonuclear leukocytes
- Bone-marrow stromal cells

---

found but one might be tempted to predict the existence of low-affinity receptors such as are found in several other lymphokines studied. Human IL-4 binds to a cell surface protein with a molecular mass of 140 kDa and to another of 70 kDa. Mouse IL-4 receptor has a molecular weight similar to the latter (Nakagima *et al.*, 1987; Park *et al.*, 1987).

The nature of the IL-5 receptors on IL-5 sensitive B-cell lines such as BCL-B20 has been examined by looking at the binding of radiolabelled recombinant eukaryotic IL-5. Despite having considerable sequence homology with IFN-γ and GM-CSF, IL-5 binds to its own surface receptor (Takatsu *et al.*, 1988). The B-cell line BCLB20 appears to express both high- and low-affinity IL-5 receptors with K_d values of 4×10^{-11} M and 1.1×10^{-9} M, respectively. There are approximately five times as many low-affinity receptors (1000 per cell) as high-affinity receptors. Very little is known about the nature of these receptors which have an apparent molecular mass of 47 kDa or the events which take place at the target-cell membrane following binding of the lymphokine.

Summary

Interleukins 4 and 5 are lymphokines produced by helper T-cells which have profound effects on the growth and differentiation of B-lymphocytes. IL-4 promotes a B-cell class switch favouring the production of IgE whereas IL-5 promotes the production of IgA. Both interleukins play a major role in the immune response towards parasitic infection and this is achieved by several mechanisms involving the production of mast cells and eosinophils. IL-4 is also a second growth factor for T-lymphocytes (TCGF-II) and is produced, in mice, by helper T-cell clones which do not produce IL-2 (TCGF-I). Both IL-4 and IL-5 are specified by genes found, in man, on chromosome 5, close to the genes for other growth factors such as IL-3 and GM-CSF. Interleukin 7 (formerly lymphopoietin-1) is a protein produced by bone marrow stromal cells which influences the proliferation of B lymphocytes precursors, IL-7 may have potential for restoring lymphocyte levels in patients whose bone marrow has been depleted by chemotherapy.

174 *Lymphokines and Interleukins*

References

Butterworth, A. E. (1984). 'Cell-mediated damage to helminths', *Adv. Parasitol.* **23**, p. 144.

Coffman, R. L. and Carty, J. (1986). 'A T-cell activity that enhances polyclonal IgE production and its inhibition by IFN-γ', *J. Immunol.* **136**, p. 949.

Coffman, R. L., Seymour, B. W. P., Lebman, D. A. *et al.* (1988). 'The role of helper T cell products in mouse B cell differentiation and isotype regulation', *Immunol. Rev.* **102**, p. 5.

Hamaguchi, Y., Hamakura, Y., Fujita, J. *et al.* (1987). 'Interleukin-4 as an essential factor for *in vitro* clonal growth of murine connective tissue-type mast cells', *J. Exp. Med.* **165**, p. 268.

Henney, C. S. (1989). 'Interleukin-7: effects on early events in lymphopoiesis', *Immunol. Today* **10**, p. 170.

Hudak, S. A., Gollnick, S. Conrad, D. H. and Kehry, M. (1987). 'Murine B-cell stimulatory factor 1 (IL-4) increases expression of the Fc receptor for IgE on normal mouse B cells', *Proc. Natl Acad. Sci. (USA)* **84**, p. 4606.

Jarret, E. E. and Miller, H. R. P. (1982). 'Production and activities of IgE in helminth infections', *Prog. Allergy* **31**, p. 178.

Kikutani, H., Suemura, M., Owaki, H. *et al.* (1986). 'Fcε receptor, a specific differentiation marker, expressed on mature B cells prior to isotype switching', *J. Exp. Med.* **164**, p. 1455.

Littman, B. H., Dastvan, F. F., Carlson, P. L. and Sanders, K. M. (1989). 'Regulation of monocytes/macrophage C2 production and HLA-DR expression by IL-4 and IFN-γ', *J. Immunol.* **142**, p. 520.

Maggi, E., Del Prete, G., Macchia, D. *et al.* (1988). 'Profiles of lymphokine activities and helper function for IgE in human T cell clones', *Eur. J. Immunol.* **18**, p. 1045.

Moller, G. (1987). 'T cell dependent and independent B cell activation', *Immunol. Rev.* **99**, pp. 5–299.

Mosmann, T. R., Cherwinski, H., Bond, M. W. *et al.* (1986). 'Two types of murine helper T cell clone. I. Definition according to profile of lymphokine activities and secreted protein', *J. Immunol.* **126**, p. 2348.

Mule, J. J., Smith, C. A. and Rosenberg, S. A. (1987). 'Interleukin-4 (B cell stimulatory factor I) can mediate the induction of lymphokine-activated killer cell activity directed against fresh tumor cells', *J. Exp. Med.* **166**, p. 792.

Nabel, G., Galli, S. J., Dvorak, A. M. *et al.* (1981). 'Inducer T lymphocytes synthesise a factor that stimulates proliferation of cloned mast cells', *Nature (London)* **291**, p. 332.

Nakagima, K., Hirano, T., Koyamo, K. and Kishimoto, T. (1987). 'Detection of receptors for murine B cell stimulatory factor 1 (BSF1): presence of functional receptors on CBA/N splenic B cells', *J. Immunol.* **139**, p. 774.

O'Garra, A., Warren, D., Holman, M. *et al.* (1986). 'Interleukin-4 (B-cell growth factor-II/eosinophil differentiation factor) is a mitogen and differentiation factor for pre-activated murine B lymphocytes'. *Proc. Natl Acad. Sci. (USA)* **83**, p. 5228.

Park, L. S., Friend, D., Sassenfeld, H. M. and Urdal, D. L. (1987). 'Characterisation of human B cell stimulatory factor 1 receptor', *J. Exp. Med.* **166**, p. 476.

Pene, J., Rousset, F., Briere, F., *et al.* (1988). 'Il-5 enhances IL-4-induced IgE production by normal human B cells. The role of soluble CD23 antigen', *Eur. J. Immunol.* **18**, p. 929.

Roitt, I. (1988). 'The acquired immune response. IV–development' in *Essential Immunology*, 6th edn, Ch. 9. Oxford, Blackwell Scientific Publications.

Sanderson, C. J., Campbell, H. D. and Young, I. G. (1988). 'Molecular and cellular biology of eosinophil differentiation factor (interleukin-5) and its effects on human and mouse B cells', *Immunol. Rev.* **102**, p. 29.

Schimpl, A. and Wecker, W. (1972). 'Replacement of T-cell function by a T-cell product', *Nature (New Biol.)* **237**, p. 15.

Sideras, P., Noma, T. and Honjo, T. (1988). 'Structure and function of interleukin 4 and 5', *Immunol. Rev.* **102**, p. 189.

Smith, C. A. S. and Rennick, D. M. (1986). 'Characterisation of a murine lymphokine distinct from IL-2 and IL-3 possessing a T cell growth factor activity and mast cell growth factor that synergises with IL-3', *Proc. Natl Acad. Sci. (USA)* **8**, p. 857.

Snapper, C. M., Finkleman, F. D. and Paul, W. E. (1988). 'Regulation of IgG_1 and IgE production by interleukin 4', *Immunol. Rev.* **102**, p. 51.

Swain, S. L., McKenzie, D. T., Dutton, R. W. *et al.* (1988). 'The role of IL-4 and IL-5: characterisation of a distinct helper T cell subset that makes IL-4 and IL-5 (Th2) and requires priming before induction of lymphokine secretion', *Immunol. Rev.* **102**, p. 77.

Takatsu, K., Tominaga, A., Harada, N. *et al.* (1988). 'T-cell-replacing factor (TRF)/interleukin 5 (IL-5): molecular and functional properties', *Immunol. Rev.* **102**, p. 10.

Yokota, T., Arai, N., De Vries, J. *et al.* (1988). 'Molecular biology of interleukin 4 and interleukin 5 genes and biology of their products that stimulate B cells, T cells and haemopoietic cells', *Immunol. Rev.* **102**, p. 137.

Zlotnik, A., Fisher, M., Roehm, N. and Zipori, D. (1987). 'Evidence for the effects of interleukin 4 (B cell stimulatory factor 1) on macrophages: enhancement of antigen-presenting ability of bone marrow-derived macrophages', *J. Immunol.* **138**, p. 4275.

8

Interleukin-6

Introduction

The previous chapter outlined the roles of interleukins 4, 5 and 7 in controlling the growth and differentiation of B-lymphocytes. Interleukin-6 (IL-6) promotes the later stages of differentiation of B-cells into plasma cells, without acting as a growth factor for stimulated B-lymphocytes. In addition, IL-6 also supports the growth of B-cell hybridomas and plasmacytomas in culture so that its presence may be useful for the production of monoclonal antibodies, especially from human hybridomas, which are often slow growing initially. Over-production of IL-6 may be implicated both in the development and symptoms of autoimmune phenomena, including those which occur in some cancer patients whose tumours produce excess of this protein.

In addition to the effects of IL-6 on B-cell differentiation, this molecule also acts on a wide range of cell types, promoting in particular the acute phase reaction to infection. IL-1 and IL-6 have almost identical effects in acute inflammatory response and synergistic responses occur in the presence of both. IL-1 is now known to promote the synthesis of IL-6 by several different cell types and it seems quite likely that several IL-1-induced activities are mediated via this molecule. Similarly, a number of cell lines which have been used as a source of IL-1 have since been found also to produce IL-6. Therefore, the results of experiments in which conditioned media from these cell lines was used as a source of IL-1 will need to be re-evaluated in the light of this knowledge.

Like most interleukins, IL-6 has appeared in the scientific literature in several guises. Its first manifestation 'in print' was in 1980 as interferon-β_2 (IFN-β_2), a molecule with weak antiviral activity produced by virus-infected fibroblasts (Weissenbach et al., 1980). Several cell types are now known to produce IL-6, including T-lymphocytes and monocytes. At the same time, the list of cells and organs which can be affected by IL-6 is long and includes B-cells, hybridomas,

Table 8.1 Alternative names for IL-6

Name	Activity promoted
IFN-β_2 (interferon-β_2)	Antiviral activity from poly(I:C)-treated fibroblasts (distinct from IFN-β)
26 kDa protein	Translation product of mRNA from fibroblasts treated with agents which induce IFN-β
BSF-2/BCDF (B-cell stimulatory factor/differentiation factor)	Increases Ab production in activated and EBV-stimulated B-cells
HPGF (hybridoma/plasmacytoma growth factor)	Supports growth of hybridomas and plasmacytomas
IL-HP1 (murine hybridoma/ plasmacytoma growth factor)	Growth factor for murine hybridomas and plasmacytomas
HSF (hepatocyte stimulating factor)	Stimulates production of acute phase proteins
TAF (T-cell activation factor)	Co-stimulates PHA-treated T-cells and thymocytes

plasmacytomas and myelomas, hepatocytes, temperature-regulatory cells in the hypothalamus, thymocytes and bone-marrow stem cells. A comprehensive list of alternative names for IL-6, together with the activities defined by them is given in Table 8.1.

IL-6 and the differentiation of B-cells

Polyclonal activation of B-lymphocytes with the Epstein–Barr virus (EBV) has provided a convenient means for stimulating the production of antibodies *in vitro* and for studying the effects of regulatory molecules on the amount and nature of the immunoglobulins produced. EBV infects B-lymphocytes and 'transforms' them so that they proliferate and develop into antibody-secreting cells. Using this system, a B-cell stimulatory factor (BSF-2), distinct from BSF-1 (IL-4) was identified in the supernatants of activated lymphocytes (Hirano *et al.*, 1986). BSF-2, now IL-6, was able to promote immunoglobulin production by EBV-transformed B-cells and, in particular, to enhance significantly the production of immunoglobulins belonging to the IgG and IgM isotypes (Fig. 8.1).

The effect of IL-6, which has also been called B-cell differentiation factor (BCDF), seems to be exerted on a terminal maturation step rather than on the activation or proliferation stages. Some evidence for this comes from experiments such as those illustrated in Fig. 8.2, in which B-cells were stimulated for 3 days with another polyclonal activator, pokeweed mitogen (PWM) in the presence of irradiated feeder cells. The addition of IL-6 on the third day resulted

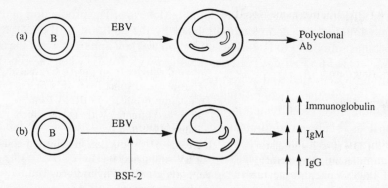

Fig. 8.1 B-cell stimulatory factor (BSF-2). Epstein–Barr virus (EBV) is a polyclonal stimulator of B-lymphocytes and EBV-transformed cells produce immunoglobulin *in vitro* (a). When BSF-2 is added to EBV-transformed cells (b) there is a significant increase in the total immunoglobulin produced and in particular, of IgM and IgG.

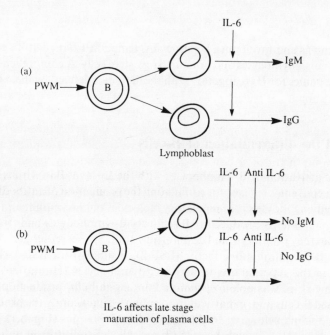

Fig. 8.2 IL-6 stimulates late maturation of plasma cells. (a) Pokeweek mitogen (PWM) is a polyclonal activator of B-lymphocytes, stimulating lymphoblast formation *in vitro*. If IL-6 is added, as much as 3 days after addition of PWM, the lymphoblasts mature into plasma cells and produce IgG and IgM. (b) The role of IL-6 is confirmed by adding an antibody to IL-6, which inhibits this differentiation, even if added up to 2 days after IL-6.

in the production by these cells of IgG and IgM *in vitro*. The production of these immunoglobulins was completely inhibited by the addition to the culture of monoclonal antibodies to IL-6. This inhibition was still apparent when the anti-IL-6 was added up to 4 days after stimulation with PWM, when the cells had already been activated and were present as large lymphoblasts. All of these findings support the viewpoint that IL-6 exerts its effects at a late stage in the maturation process of B-lymphocytes into plasma cells (Muraguchi *et al.*, 1988).

IL-6 does not appear to stimulate the proliferation of activated B-cells but acts entirely as a differentiation factor. However, IL-6 is known to synergize with IL-1 in promoting the growth of B-cells which have already been activated (Wong and Clark, 1988). For example, murine IL-6, which on its own is a poor stimulator of B-cells activated with anti-immunoglobulin, synergizes with IL-1 to induce good proliferation of such lymphocytes. IL-6 and IL-1 may also induce some limited proliferation in freshly isolated populations of 'normal' lymphocytes although it is assumed that the cells which respond have been activated *in vivo* by natural infection. The minimal growth-promoting activity on resting B-cells of IL-6 *per se* is in direct contrast with its known effects in stimulating the growth of hybridomas and plasmacytomas.

Hybridoma/plasmacytoma growth factor (HPGF)

IL-6 is a potent growth factor for plasmacytomas or myelomas which are malignant tumours of plasma cell origin. As might be expected from their origin, these tumour cells secrete homogeneous antibody, the specificity of which is seldom indentified. Under 'normal' circumstances, the development of a plasma-acytoma is a rare event which, when it occurs, usually takes place within the bone marrow. In rodents, however, it has been found that myelomas can be induced in mice which have been injected with mineral oil via the intraperitonal route (Potter and Boyce, 1962). The mineral oil-induced plasmacytoma (MOPC) grows initially as a suspension of malignant cells in the peritoneal fluid, forming an 'ascites' fluid which is rich in myeloma cells.

MOPC are frequently used as fusion partners for B-cells for the production of hybridomas making monoclonal antibodies, and for this technique it is absolutely necessary that they grow well in tissue culture. However, although myeloma cells grow extremely well in the peritoneal fluid of the animal in which they were raised, adaptation, it appears, is dependent on the presence, at least in the first instance, of irradiated feeder cells, such as peripheral blood leukocytes. Similarly, B-cell hybridomas, produced by the fusion of antibody-producing spleen cells with myelomas, are also frequently dependent in the initial stages, on the presence of irradiated leukocytes for successful growth *in vitro*.

In the same way that haemopoietic colony stimulating factors were discovered by analysing the conditioned media of cells used for feeder layers in bone-marrow stem-cell cultures, it was discovered that supernatants from irradiated feeder cells, and particularly of monocytes and T-cells, could to some extent substitute for the cells themselves in supporting the growth of hybridomas or plasmacytomas. In 1987, human fibroblasts treated with IL-1 or synthetic double-stranded polyribonucleotides such as poly(rI:rC) (polyinosinic–polycytidylic acid) were found to produce a potent hybridoma/plasmacytoma growth factor (HPGF) (Van Damme *et al.*, 1987). Similar conditions had, some years earlier, been found to stimulate the production by fibroblasts of a novel interferon, IFN-β_2. The murine equivalent of HPGF, which is induced under essentially similar conditions, and has almost identical activities, was known initially as interleukin-HP1 (IL-HP1). This molecule has structural similarities to HPGF and is the murine equivalent of IL-6. IL-6 can be produced by a variety of human and murine cells following treatment with IL-1 or TNF, and this has been measured by the ability of supernatants from these cells to act as HPGF. The list of cells which can produce HPGF include macrophages, T-cells, fibroblasts, endothelial cells and MG-63, a human cell line derived from an osteosarcoma.

The growth-promoting ability of IL-6 on hybridomas and plasmacytomas is in contrast with its effect on B-cells where it stimulates differentiation rather than growth. IL-6 can, however, act as a co-stimulator of proliferation by synergizing, for example with IL-1. Differential effects may be related to both the level of expression of cell receptors for IL-6 and the affinity of these receptors, about which much more needs to be known.

IL-6 and the acute phase response

Interleukin-6 is an important mediator of the acute phase response along with IL-1 and TNF (Gauldie *et al.*, 1987). IL-6 has been found to be identical to hepatocyte-stimulating factor (HSF), a product of activated macrophages discovered in 1983, which was shown to stimulate the synthesis of fibrinogen by rat hepatoma cells. When recombinant human IL-6 is injected into rats there is an increase in the blood levels of all the acute phase proteins and this increase is both rapid in onset and dose-dependent (Geiger *et al.*, 1988). At the same time IL-6 causes a dose-dependent decrease in the amount of albumin synthesized by the liver. Maximum levels of mRNA specifying acute phase proteins can be found in hepatocytes at 4 h after injection of IL-6. IL-1 is known to induce the synthesis of IL-6 in several cell types so that the extent to which IL-1 induces the acute phase response by itself or through the induction of IL-6 is not yet fully understood; most likely it does both. Recombinant IL-6 induces the synthesis of all the major acute phase proteins and this can be inhibited by a monoclonal antibody to IL-6. A comparison between the effects of IL-1, IL-6 and TNF on the induction of acute phase proteins by human hepatoma cells in culture has shown that all three molecules produce comparable stimulation of acute phase proteins *in vitro*, both in terms of the types of proteins stimulated and inhibited, and the kinetics of the response (Ramadori *et al.*, 1988). Analysis of the effects of these

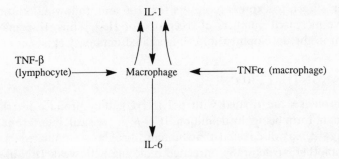

Fig. 8.3 IL-6 and the acute phase response. TNF-α (macrophage-derived) and TNF-β (lymphocyte-derived), both stimulate the production of IL-1 by macrophages. IL-1 in turn stimulates the production of IL-6 which mediates many of the effects of these molecules in inducing the acute phase response.

three molecules on the acute phase response is made more complicated by the fact that, while IL-1 induces the synthesis of IL-6 in target cells, TNF can also stimulate the production of IL-1 (Fig. 8.3).

The acute phase response is not simply marked by an increase in acute phase proteins. One other, readily quantifiable feature of the acute response is the rapid onset of fever which is also induced by IL-6. Whereas TNF causes a biphasic fever since it has direct and indirect pyrogenic activity (the indirect occurring via IL-1), the fever which is induced by IL-6 is, like IL-1, monophasic and the kinetics of the induction of fever by IL-6 are identical to IL-1.

IL-6 and haemopoiesis

Both human and murine IL-6 support the growth of granulocyte/monocyte precursors from mouse bone marrow but neither has this effect with human bone marrow stem cells. However, IL-6 from both species is able to synergize with IL-3 in supporting the proliferation of bone marrow stem cells in culture. The effect of IL-6 in concert with IL-3 is to increase the number of stem-cell colonies produced from a given number of bone marrow cells. IL-6 is thought to render stem cells more responsive to IL-3 possibly by triggering 'resting' stem cells so that they enter into the cell cycle (Ikebuchi *et al.*, 1987). It follows that if stem cells divide more frequently, there are more progeny which can be triggered into differentiation by IL-3, the pan-specific haemopoietin or the multi-CSF.

IL-6 AND T-LYMPHOCYTES

When fibroblasts are treated with IL-1, they release a factor which co-stimulates thymocytes treated with PHA. The activity is now known to be due to IL-6. Pure IL-6 also synergizes with IL-1 in the co-stimulation assay. Resting lymphocytes have been shown to express receptors for IL-6 and, following treatment with IL-6, have increased numbers of receptors for IL-2. Thus, IL-6 may also be important in the development of cell-mediated immunity (Elias *et al.*, 1989).

IS IL-6 AN INTERFERON?

When fibroblasts are treated with poly(rI:rC), they produce interferon, the predominant form being, by definition, IFN-β, a 'classical' interferon. Almost a decade ago it was discovered that human fibroblasts stimulated in this way released another, structurally unrelated molecule with weak IFN-like activity which became known as IFN-β_2. An antiserum prepared against IFN-β was said to neutralize the activity of this 'novel' interferon, but this finding still remains to be explained. There is minimal amino acid homology between the IFN-β and IFN-β_2 and an antiserum to IFN-β does not precipitate IFN-β_2 as might be expected if similar epitopes were found on the two molecules. In 1982, mRNA isolated from stimulated fibroblasts and translated in *Xenopus* oocytes was shown to give rise to a 26 kDa protein with interferon-like activity. More recently, cDNA complementary to RNA specifying the 26 kDa protein was shown to hybridize with the human HPGF, to which it is now known to be identical.

The antiviral activity of IFN-β_2 has been a subject of much speculation and controversy. While some immunologists have been unable to demonstrate antiviral factors distinct from IFN-β in poly(rI:rC) fibroblasts, others have produced evidence to support its existence. From the latter, it is evident that the activity of IFN-β_2 is weak compared with the classical interferons, and specific activities (units of activity per mg of protein) between 10^4 and 10^5 times lower than the classical interferons have been quoted. Neutralization of an interferon by antibody to a structurally unrelated molecule is, however, quite hard to explain, particularly since the precipitation tests reveal no shared epitopes (Billiau, 1987; Hirano *et al.*, 1988).

Production of IL-6

IL-6 was initially purified from fibroblasts stimulated with poly(rI:rC). Several human cell lines constitutively produce human IL-6 and these include some T-cell lines derived from patients with adult T-cell leukaemia, the human bladder carcinoma cell line T24, and cells derived from cardiac myxoma, a tumour which grows within the atrium of the heart. In all these cells, IL-6 production appears to be dysregulated.

Many different cell types produce IL-6 after stimulation with IL-1 and/or TNF, including fibroblasts, endothelial cells and the MG-63 osteosarcoma cell line. Recombinant IL-6 is also now available commercially, with high specific activities in hybridoma stimulation or other assay systems.

Assays for IL-6

The problem of finding a specific bioassay for a given lymphokine is becoming more difficult with the recognition that most of these molecules have overlapping activities. IL-6 is no exception since many of its activities overlap with TNF and, particularly, IL-1. For example, IL-1 has commonly been assayed by its ability to co-stimulate thymocytes in the presence of PHA but IL-6 is also active in this assay. Moreover, several of the activities of IL-1 can be attributed to its effects in inducing the synthesis of IL-6. In such cases, a more specific assay would be required or, at the least, controls should include additions of monoclonal antibodies to IL-6 or IL-1 in the incubation mixture. IL-6 can be measured by its growth effect on a murine hybridoma line, B9. This assay is said to be specific for IL-6 and has a sensitivity for both human and murine IL-6 of around 5×10^{-13} g IL-6/ml (Helle *et al.*, 1988).

Recently, an ELISA assay was designed which used recombinant human IL-6 and a monoclonal antibody prepared in mice. Several hybridomas produced a satisfactory monoclonal antibody but one successful hybridoma also became dependent on IL-6 for continued growth. This cell line can be used to assay for IL-6 because 10^{-12} g quantities of IL-6 can stimulate growth. In addition, the monoclonal antibody which this hybridoma produces has been used to establish an ELISA assay for IL-6 with similar sensitivity (Matsuda *et al.*, 1988).

Molecular biology

The genes for human and murine IL-6 have both been cloned in recent years. Complementary DNA for human IL-6 specifies a single polypeptide chain having 212 amino acid residues, including a signal sequence of 28 hydrophobic residues which is cleaved prior to secretion. Secreted human IL-6 therefore has a molecular weight of 26 kDa and contains 184 amino acid residues. The mature molecule is N-glycosylated at two sites. There is some limited amino acid sequence homology between human IL-6 and human G-CSF which also have a similar gene organization, indicating that they may be descended from a common ancestral gene. Both genes have 5 exons, the sizes being identical between the two molecules. The gene for human IL-6 is unusual in that it has several different sites at which transcription can be initiated. Since a number of different cell types are able to secrete IL-6, there is the possibility that cells of different histogenic origin may use different sites. The significance, though, still remains to be seen (Yasukawa *et al.*, 1987).

An initial and limited sequence analysis of the amino terminus of the murine hybridoma growth factor, IL-HP1 rather surprisingly revealed that its amino terminal amino acid sequence was totally dissimilar from that of the human hybridoma/plasmacytoma growth factor. IL-HP1 not only has a similar spectrum of activity to human IL-6 but its synthesis in murine T-cells, macrophages and endothelial cells is induced under very similar circumstances. It has since transpired that, while there is no homology in the amino terminus, murine and human IL-6 have 42% homology at the amino acid level over the entire polypeptide sequence (and 65% at the DNA level). IL-6 is not species-specific and human IL-6 stimulates murine cells and vice versa.

The entire sequence of murine IL-HP1 was determined by prediction from the cDNA sequence (Van Snick *et al.*, 1988). Polyadenylated RNA was isolated from stimulated cells and used to prepare a cDNA library. An oligonucleotide probe was constructed which was complementary to the amino terminal sequence of IL-HP1 purified from helper T-cell clones and subjected to limited sequence analysis (Fig. 8.4). Murine IL-HP1 has 212 amino acids including a signal peptide of 24 hydrophobic residues, the remaining residues giving it a molecular

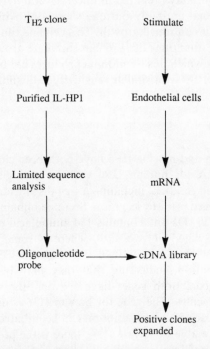

Fig. 8.4   Cloning of murine IL-HP1 (mouse IL-6). IL-HP1 was extensively purified from the culture supernatants of T_{H2} clones and subjected to limited N-terminal sequence analysis. Knowing the sequence of a short peptide at the N-terminus allowed the synthesis of a complementary oligonucleotide probe. IL-6 producing cells were stimulated appropriately and newly synthesized mRNA extracted and used to construct a cDNA library. The library was probed with the synthetic oligonucleotide probe, to determine the clone with IL-HP1-specific DNA.

mass of almost 22 kDa. Four cysteine molecules are found in both the human and murine IL-6. These cysteines are essential for biological activity which is greatly diminished following reduction and alkylation. IL-HP1 has several potential O-glycosylation sites, and glycosylation may increase this mass up to 29 kDa. Differing degrees of glycosylation may affect the binding of IL-6 to receptors on different cells and this may account for the differing activities induced in different cell types. High-affinity IL-6 receptors are widely distributed on cells including haemopoietic cells and activated B-cells. The wide range of activity *in vivo* must indicate a similarly wide range of receptor-positive cells. It might be expected, for example, that cells in the temperature regulatory centre in the brain will have such receptors.

Immunopathology and IL-6

The dysregulation of IL-6 production has been seen in several pathological situations although direct evidence that this is a cause rather than an effect can be difficult to obtain. Pathological situations in which IL-6 levels are elevated include infections with retroviruses such as HIV and HTLV-I (see below), some autoimmune diseases such as rheumatoid arthritis, and in patients with certain types of benign or malignant tumour where production of IL-6 by the tumour is associated with autoimmune manifestations. There is also evidence to suggest that over-production of IL-6 may be related to the development of myelomas *in vivo*.

IL-6 AND THE DEVELOPMENT OF MYELOMAS

IL-6 is a potent growth factor for hybridomas and myelomas *in vitro*. Peritoneal macrophages of mice which have been injected with mineral oil to promote the production of a myeloma have been found to secrete large amounts of IL-6, as do local granulomas induced in the peritoneum by this treatment. The fact that mineral oil consistently produces myeloma, and that this is related to high IL-6 levels, has led to the idea that the 'natural' development of at least some myelomas may be the result of dysregulation of IL-6 rather than of immunoglobulin (Kawano *et al.*, 1988). Moreover, the freshly isolated myeloma cells of a significant number of patients produce IL-6, have receptors for IL-6, and are stimulated into growth by the presence of IL-6. Thus, the continued proliferation of myeloma cells *in vivo* may be the result of an autocrine stimulation (Fig. 8.5). If this is the case, the administration of monoclonal antibodies to IL-6 might break this stimulatory cycle. Alternatively, toxic chemicals could be targetted at myeloma cells by a monoclonal antibody against the IL-6 receptor.

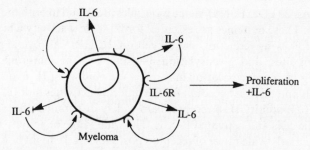

Fig. 8.5 Autocrine stimulation of myeloma cells. Fresh myeloma cells from several patients were shown both to express IL-6 receptors and to produce IL-6 *in vitro*. One recent suggestion for the development of myelomas *in vivo* suggests an autocrine role for IL-6 in which an aberrant production of IL-6 by these cells causes further proliferation.

IL-6 AND RETROVIRUSES

The human immunodeficiency virus, HIV, infects helper T-cells which are subsequently destroyed, leaving an immune deficit which results, ultimately, in AIDS. Paradoxically, immunoglobulin levels in patients infected with HIV are frequently elevated above normal and this is due to polyclonal activation of B-lymphocytes. Several explanations have been suggested for this phenomenon, including reactivation of latent EBV due to generalized immunosuppression and infection of B-cells with HIV, even though they lack the CD4 protein which acts as the cellular receptor for the virus. Recently, it has been shown that exposure of peripheral blood mononuclear cells to HIV promotes the production of IL-6 by monocytes and that this occurs even in the absence of T-lymphocytes. This IL-6 may then promote the terminal maturation of activated B-cells transformed by latent EBV. The Epstein–Barr virus is latent in a very high proportion of humans, having been acquired, usually, in childhood (Makajima *et al.*, 1989).

HTLV-I (human lymphotropic virus I) is another retrovirus which infects human CD4[+] cells. HTLV-I infection is responsible for the development of adult T-cell leukaemia (ATL) rather than cytolysis of infected cells. Lymphocyte cell lines derived from patients with ATL produce numerous lymphokines *in vitro* including GM-CSF, IL-5 and IL-6, as well as expressing abnormally high levels of the low affinity IL-2 receptor (Yoshida and Seike, 1987). The HTLV-I virus contains a gene which codes for a protein which regulates lymphokine genes and which, if transferred to other cells by transfection, can stimulate the production of lymphokines in these cells. The isolation of a viral regulatory protein may provide a means of attacking the disease if the abnormal levels of lymphokines are important in the uncontrolled proliferation which results in leukaemia. Moreover, such a regulatory gene may be useful for stimulating the production of lymphokines in culture, and perhaps in the recognition of new lymphokine activities.

IL-6 AND AUTOIMMUNITY

IL-6, along with many other lymphokines, has been implicated in the development of rheumatoid arthritis (RA) (Kishimoto and Hirano, 1988). The synovial fluids from affected joints in these patients have been shown to contain a factor which promotes immunoglobulin secretion in activated B-lymphocytes. High levels of IL-6 have been found in the synovial fluids of a high proportion (88%) of patients with RA and this correlates with both an increase in acute phase proteins and elevation of immunoglobulin levels in the blood due to polyclonal activation of B-cells. The synovial tissues of RA patients are frequently infiltrated with plasma cells producing antibody locally. This plasma-cell infiltrate may be the result of local IL-6 production causing differentiation of activated B-cells locally.

Castleman's disease is characterized by chronic swelling of lymph nodes which are infiltrated with plasma cells. The patients have elevated levels of plasma immunoglobulins and acute phase proteins in addition to fever. Surgical removal of the affected lymph nodes produces almost immediate improvements in the systemic symptons (Keller *et al.*, 1972). When cells from affected nodes are cultured, they release IL-6 constitutively so that dysregulation of IL-6 again seems to be strongly implicated in the development of this disease.

A number of tumours secrete large amounts of IL-6 and patients with these tumours develop autoimmune symptoms. Cardiac myxoma is a benign tumour which develops in the atrium in the heart. Almost a third of patients with cardiac myxoma in one study had autoantibodies in their blood (Hirano *et al.*, 1987). Similar, if less frequent, findings have occurred in some patients with cervical cancer. In these cases, surgical removal of the tumour also results in alleviation of the autoimmunity.

Summary

Although IL-6 has only recently been cloned, it has proved to have remarkably widespread effects on cells directly and indirectly involved with the immune system. Its activity as a B-cell differentiation factor and co-stimulator of B-cells makes it important in the development of primary and secondary immune responses where IgG and IgM are the principal antibodies. Its activity in co-stimulating the proliferation of thymocytes and T-lymphocytes in the presence of sub-optimal concentrations of PHA may indicate that it is also important in the development of cell-mediated immunity. In addition, IL-6 promotes IL-3-induced haemopoiesis which may be significant in haemopoiesis induced by infection.

IL-6 also forms part of the first defence mechanism against infection: it is one of the three modulators of the acute phase response, stimulating the production of proteins with direct or indirect antibacterial effects. In addition, its interferon activity (which is disputed) may constitute a first-line defence against viruses. Indications that IL-6 is involved in the development of autoimmune symptoms and myeloma, may lead to new approaches to the treatment of these diseases.

References

Billiau, A. (1987). 'Interferon β_2 as a promoter of growth and differentiation of B cells', *Immunol. Today* **8**, p. 84.

Elias, J. A., Trinchieri, G., Beck, J. M. *et al.* (1989). 'A synergistic interaction of IL-6 and IL-1 mediates the thymocyte-stimulating activity produced by rIL-1-stimulated fibroblasts', *J. Immunol.* **142**, p. 509.

Gauldie, J., Richards, C., Harnish, D. *et al.* (1987). 'Interferon $\beta2$/BSF2 shares identity with monocyte-derived hepatocyte-stimulating factor (HSF) and regulates the major acute phase protein response in liver cells', *Proc. Natl Acad. Sci. (USA)* **84**, p. 7251.

Geiger, T., Andus, T., Klapproth, J. *et al.* (1988). 'Induction of rat acute-phase protein by IL-6 *in vivo*', *Eur. J. Biochem.* **175**, p. 181.

Hirano, T., Yasukawa, K., Harade, H. *et al.* (1986). 'Complementary DNA for a novel human interleukin (BSF-2) that induces B lymphocytes to produce immunoglobulin', *Nature (London)* **324**, p. 73.

Hirano, T., Taga, T. Yasukawa, K. *et al.* (1987). 'Human B cell differentiation factor defined by an anti-peptide antibody and its possible role in autoantibody production', *Proc. Natl Acad. Sci. (USA)* **84**, p. 228.

Hirano, T., Matsuda, T., Hosoi, K. *et al.* (1988). 'Absence of antiviral activity in recombinant B cell stimulatory factor-2 (BSF-2)', *Immunol. Lett.* **17**, p. 41.

Helle, M., Brakenhoff, J. P., De-Groot, E. R. and Aarden, L. A. (1988). 'IL-6 is involved in IL-1-induced activities', *Eur. J. Immunol.* **18**, p. 957.

Ikebuchi, K., Wong, G. G., Clark, S. C. *et al.* (1987). 'Interleukin-6 enhancement of interleukin-3-dependent proliferation of multipotential haemopoietic progenitors', *Proc. Natl Acad. Sci. (USA)* **84**, p. 9035.

Kishimoto, T. and Hirano, T. (1988). 'A new interleukin with pleiotropic activities', *Bioessays* **9**, p. 11.

Keller, A. R., Hochholtzer, L. and Castleman, B. (1972). 'Hyalin-vascular and plasma-cell types of giant lymph node hyperplasia of the mediastinum and other locations', *Cancer* **29**, p. 670.

Kawano, M., Hirano, T., Masuda, T. *et al.* (1988). 'Autocrine generation and requirement of BSF-2/IL-6 for human multiple myelomas', *Nature* **332**, p. 83.

Makajima, K., Martinez-Maza, O., Hirano, T. *et al.* (1989). 'Induction of interleukin-6 by the human immunodeficiency virus (HIV)', *J. Immunol.* **142**, p. 531.

Matsuda, T., Hirano, T. and Kishimoto, T. (1988). 'Establishment of an interleukin-6 (IL-6)/B cell stimulatory factor-2-dependent cell line and preparation of anti-IL-6 monoclonal antibodies', *Eur. J. Immunol.* **18**, p. 951.

Muraguchi, A., Hirano, T., Tang, B. *et al.* (1988). 'The essential role of B cell stimulatory factor-2 (BSF-2/IL-6) for the terminal differentiation of B cells', *J. Exp. Med.* **167**, p. 332.

Potter, M. and Boyce, C. (1962). 'Induction of plasma cell neoplasms in strain Balb/C mice with mineral oil and mineral oil adjuvants', *Nature (London)* **193**, p. 1086.

Ramadori, G., Van Damme, J., Rieder, H. and Meyer, zum Buschenfelde, K-H. (1988). 'IL-6, the third mediator of acute phase reactions, modulates hepatic protein synthesis in humans and the mouse. Comparison with IL-1β and TNFα', *Eur. J. Immunol.* **18**, p. 1259.

Van Damme, J., Opdenakker, G., Simpson, R. J. *et al.* (1987). 'Identification of the human 26-kD protein, interferon $\beta2$ (IFN-$\beta2$) as a hybridoma/plasmacytoma growth factor induced by interleukin-1 and tumour necrosis factor', *J. Exp. Med.* **165**, p. 914.

Van Snick, J., Cayphas, S., Szikora, J.-P. *et al.* (1988). 'cDNA cloning of murine interleukin-HP1: homology with human interleukin-6', *Eur. J. Immunol.* **18**, p. 193.

Vink, A., Goulie, P. G. Wauters, P. *et al.* (1988). 'B cell growth and differentiation activity of interleukin HP1 and related murine plasmacytoma growth factors. Synergy with IL-1', *Eur. J. Immunol.* **18**, p. 607.

Weissenbach, J., Chernajovsky, Y., Zeevi, M. *et al.* (1980). 'Two interferon mRNAs in human fibroblasts: *in vitro* translation and *Escherichia coli* cloning studies', *Proc. Natl Acad. Sci. (USA)* **77**, p. 7152.

Wong, G. C. and Clark, S. C. (1988). 'Multiple actions of interleukin-6 within a cytokine network', *Immunol. Today* **9**, p. 137.

Yasukawa, K., Hirano, T., Watanabe, Y. *et al.* (1987). 'Structure and expression of human B cell stimulatory factor 2 (BSF-2/IL-6) gene', *EMBO J.* **6**, p. 2939.

Yoshida, M. and Seike, M. (1987). 'Recent advances in the molecular biology of HTLV-1: transactivation of viral and cellular genes', *Ann. Rev. Immunol.* **5**, p. 541.

9

Interferon-γ

Introduction

People who have an active viral infection are commonly resistant to infection with another virus, and this phenomenon is known as viral 'interference'. Jenner first described viral interference in 1804 when he recorded that some patients with active herpes virus infection did not develop the usual 'pox' lesion after immunization with the vaccinia virus. One hundred and fifty years later (Isaacs and Lindenmann, 1957), viral interference was attributed to a soluble product released by the infected cells. Isaacs and Lindenmann first coined the term 'interferon' when they showed that the supernatants from fragments of chick choriollantoic membrane infected with influenza virus contained a factor which would interfere with viral infection of other cells.

An interferon (IFN) is now defined by the Interferon Nomenclature Committee 1980 (Stewart *et al.*, 1980) as a protein which 'exerts virus-non-specific antiviral activity at least in homologous cells through cellular metabolic processes involving synthesis of both RNA and protein'. Thus, IFNs exert an indirect antiviral activity by inducing genes whose products inhibit viral replication (Fig. 9.1) and IFN-γ is only one of several molecules which fit this criterion.

In the 1970s, IFNs were shown to cause the regression of some established tumours in animals and, later, in humans (Gresser and Bourali-Mauri, 1972). In addition, interferon inhibited the proliferation of tumour cells *in vitro*. The appearance of any new 'drug' with antitumour properties always provokes a great deal of research and media interest and interferons were no exception. The research explosion which ensued culminated in extensive clinical trials which have produced many disappointments as well as one or two rather unexpected bonuses. However, the great attention shown to the growth regulatory properties of interferons generally has served also to encourage scientists to re-examine the antiviral properties. As yet, there is no universal 'antibiotic' for viral infection

Virus-infected cells

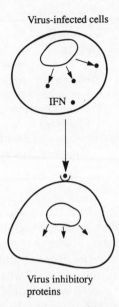

IFN •

Virus inhibitory
proteins

Fig. 9.1 Antiviral activity of interferon (IFN). Virus-infected cells secrets interferon which binds to specific receptors on other cells, and induces the production by these cells of proteins which inhibit the replication of viruses. Thus, active viral infection, inducing the production of IFN, can protect an individual against infection with a second, unrelated virus.

and the most effective antiviral drugs, the nucleoside analogues, have toxic effects on those tissues which have a high cellular turnover. An efficacious and non-toxic antiviral agent such as IFN, which could be used prophylactically for a variety of viral infections from the common cold to viral hepatitis or even human immunodeficiency virus (HIV), would have enormous clinical and commercial potential.

Classification of interferons

IFNs belong to one of two major 'types' as defined by several criteria (Table 9.1), the major differences between these two types being the nature of the inducing agent and of the producing cell. Classical or Type-I IFNs are secreted by all nucleated cells following infection with a virus. Type-I IFNs belong to one of two subtypes, interferons α and β (IFN-α and IFN-β), based on structural differences which can be detected serologically (that is, with specific antibodies). Although most nucleated cells produce IFN-α and IFN-β when infected with a virus, they are the predominant types produced by virus-infected leukocytes and fibroblasts,

Table 9.1   Classification of interferons

Interferon family	Type	Definition
IFN-α	I	Predominant form produced by virus-infected leukocytes
IFN-β	I	Predominant form produced by virus-infected fibroblasts
IFN-γ	II	'Immune'; produced by antigen- or mitogen-stimulated T-cells

respectively. In 1965, a third IFN-like activity was discovered in the supernatants of lymphocytes stimulated with phytohaemagglutinin (PHA) (Wheelock, 1965). This molecule however was found to differ in several ways from the α and β forms both in the stimulus for its release, its structure and physico-chemical properties, and in its range of activities, only some of which overlap with those of the classical interferons. 'Immune' or Type-II interferon is now most commonly known as interferon-γ (IFN-γ). IFN-γ is a true lymphokine, being the product of lymphocytes activated with specific antigens or lectins. For this reason, the remainder of this chapter will focus on IFN-γ which apart from its antiviral activity is a potent modulator of immune responses. IFN-γ has multiple effects on cells of the immune system and this immunomodulatory role may be more significant *in vivo* than its antiviral activity. None the less, both IFN-α and IFN-β do have some immunomodulatory and growth-regulatory properties which they share with IFN-γ and these will be discussed where appropriate. In addition to IFNs there is another molecule with interferon-like antiviral activity, which was originally called IFN-β_2. IFN-β_2 was discovered in the supernatants of fibroblasts under conditions in which they produce classical IFN-β. IFN-β_2 has now been shown to be identical to IL-6, which is discussed in Chapter 8 but its supposed interferon-like activity is disputed (Billiau, 1987).

Cellular origin of IFN-γ

T-LYMPHOCYTES

These are the major producers of IFN-γ *in vivo*. Production can be induced *in vitro* by stimulating T-cells from 'immune' animals with the specific antigen. Alternatively, polyclonal activation of T-cells with PHA or with anti-CD3 (Van Wauwe *et al.*, 1980) antibodies results in the release of IFN-γ into the culture media. Both helper (CD4[+]) and cytotoxic (CD8[+]) T-cells have the capacity to produce IFN-γ and indeed do so after activation with anti-CD3. However, it is likely that the helper cell is the main producer. The release of IL-2 by T_H seems to be the main stimulus for the sequential synthesis of IFN-γ and other lymphokines

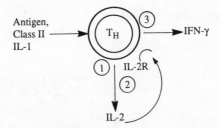

Fig. 9.2 Release of IFN-γ by helper T-lymphocytes. Stimulation of T$_H$ by specific antigen complexed on the surface of an antigen-presenting cell with Class II MHC molecules, stimulates the release of IL-2 (1) and the expression of high-affinity IL-2 receptors (2). The IL-2 then stimulates the release of other lymphokines, including IFN-γ in an autocrine fashion (3).

(Fig. 9.2) (Kronke *et al.*, 1985). When exogenous IL-2 is added to lymphocytes in culture, there is a significant increase in the amount of IFN-γ released and this release can be inhibited by the addition of monoclonal antibodies specific for the IL-2 receptor (Anti-Tac) (Kasahara *et al.*, 1983).

LARGE GRANULAR LYMPHOCYTES (LGL)

These constitute a second source of IFN-γ *in vivo*. The LGL fraction of human blood contains cells with natural killer (NK) activity which is directed in a non-specific manner against tumour cells and virus-infected cells. When LGL are treated with IL-2, they release IFN-γ in addition to more IL-2. The release of IFN-γ by these cells accounts in part for the increase in cytotoxicity of these cells after they have been incubated with IL-2 (Trinchieri *et al.*, 1984; Sandvig *et al.*, 1987). The production of IFN-γ by LGL has been demonstrated in studies such as that illustrated in Fig. 9.3, in which peripheral blood mononuclear cells were stimulated with anti-CD3 antibodies. When the cells producing IFN-γ were characterized, it was shown that approximately half of the IFN-γ was the product of CD4$^+$ and CD8$^+$ cells. NK cells constituted a small proportion of the remainder, with a large proportion being produced by cells positive for the monocyte marker, OKM1, but lacking in major histocompatibility complex (MHC) Class II antigens (Andersson *et al.*, 1986).

Multiple activities of IFN-γ

IFN-γ exerts multiple effects on a variety of cells of the immune system and a list of these activities is shown in Table 9.2. Some of these activities are common to interferons of all types but some are unique to IFN-γ. It should already by evident from previous chapters that the idea of synergism between lymphokines

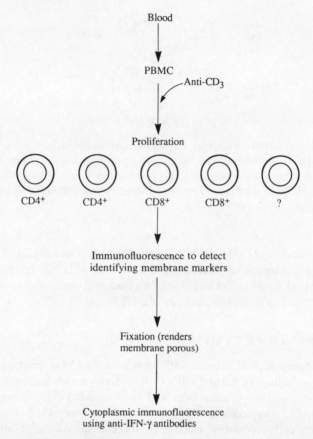

Fig. 9.3 Investigation of IFN-γ-producing cells. Peripheral blood mononuclear cells (PBMC) were isolated from whole blood by centrifugation on Ficoll/Triosil gradients. Incubation with the monoclonal antibody, anti-CD3, stimulates proliferation of all cells bearing the CD3 marker, i.e. T-cells. The proliferating cells were identified by immunofluorescence using a panel of monoclonal antibodies. The same cells were then fixed and a monoclonal antibody used to detect cytoplasmic IFN-γ by immunofluorescence. In this way, it was established that both T_c and T_H can produce IFN-γ.

is of great current interest. IFN-γ exerts synergistic effects with several other proteins such as tumour necrosis factors α and β (TNF-α/β) (in antiviral immunity and in the up-regulation of MHC antigens). The overlapping activities exhibited by several lymphokines are reflected in the overlapping nature of the polypeptides which are induced by them (Beresini *et al.*, 1988). However, IFN-γ can also oppose the effects of other lymphokines as, for example, in its inhibition of the IL-4 induced production of IgE.

Table 9.2 Biological properties of IFN-γ

Action of IFN-γ	Target cell
Inhibits viral replication	All nucleated cells tested
Inhibits growth of cells	Normal and tumour cells *in vitro*
Promotes cell differentiation	Cultured HL60 myelomonocytic cells
Increases MHC expression	All nucleated cells (Class I); macrophages, monocytes, other APC, B-cells, endothelial cells (Class II)
Increases phagocytosis	Macrophages (macrophage activation factor, MAF)
Increases cytotoxicity	Macrophages, monocytes, natural killer cells, cytotoxic T-cells
Increases antibody production	Plasma cells
Decreases antibody production	Proliferating B-cells

ANTIVIRAL ACTIVITY

Interferon-γ, by definition, possesses antiviral activity. Like the classical interferons IFN-γ is secreted by a cell after appropriate stimulation, and binds to cell surface receptors on adjacent, non-infected cells. Following binding, it promotes a number of activities of which the following enzymes are appropriate to antiviral immunity.

Protein kinase

All interferons induce the synthesis of a protein kinase in target cells. This enzyme phosphorylates, and therefore inactivates, the eukaryotic initiation factor (eIF-2), a protein which is essential to the first stages of protein synthesis. Thus, any virus-directed protein synthesis, for example, the synthesis of new viral capsids (protein coats) is inhibited.

2′5′-Polyadenylate synthetase (2–5A)

This is an enzyme which stimulates the conversion of ATP to 2′5′-polyadenylate polymers which indirectly bring about the degradation of viral mRNA by activating an endonuclease.

Both these enzyme activities are induced by IFNs of all classes but the effectiveness of either in mediating antiviral activity is uncertain. Both enzymes require the presence of double-stranded RNA for full activity and it is sometimes difficult to see where this would come from in terms of IFN-γ which is induced by specific antigen and not by viruses (Czarniecki *et al.*, 1984).

INHIBITION OF CELL GROWTH

All interferons have growth-inhibitory properties with IFN-γ having the highest activity in this respect (Rubin and Gupta, 1980). The effects of IFN-γ depend partly on the sensitivity of the target cell. Thus, while most cells are simply prevented from growing (cytostasis), others are destroyed (cytocidal action). In particular, IFN-γ has been shown to be cytocidal towards cultured transformed cells such as HeLa cells. However, some of these direct cytolytic effects of IFN-γ on tumour cells, which held out so much hope for tumour therapy, have more recently been attributed to contamination of the semi-pure preparations with TNF (see Chapter 10). In support of this is the finding that recombinant TNF and IFN-γ have synergistic cytolytic effects *in vitro*. The growth-inhibitory effects of all interferons can in part be explained by the induction of 2–5A and protein kinase and their subsequent effects on protein synthesis. IFN-treated cells also express fewer receptors for transferrin in the cell membrane and this in itself may result in cytostasis. Of course, the bulk of the investigations on this effect of IFNs, in general, has been aimed at inhibiting the growth of tumours in humans. In the last six years or so, IFN-γ has been used extensively in clinical trials, many of which are still ongoing.

REGULATION OF CELL DIFFERENTIATION

As well as inhibiting the growth of cells, IFNs can also promote cell differentiation and increase the expression of a differentiated function. This is exemplified by the up-regulation of MHC antigens and by the increase in the cytotoxicity of NK cells and specific cytotoxic T-lymphocytes following incubation with IFN. IFN-γ may also have a role in haemopoiesis since it can stimulate the differentiation of pro-myelomonocytic cells *in vitro*. For example, HL60 is an established human pro-myelomonocytic leukaemic line which can be induced by a variety of stimuli to develop into either monocytes or granulocytes. IFN-γ (Fig. 9.4) promotes monocyte differentiation. Type-I IFN does not have this property (Ball *et al.,* 1984).

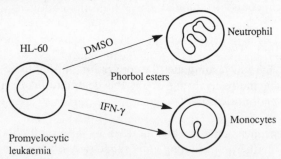

Fig. 9.4   IFN-γ and monocyte differentiation. HL-60 is a pro-myelomonocytic leukaemia which can be induced to differentiate into either neutrophils or monocytes. Dimethylsulphoxide (DMSO) stimulates neutrophil differentiation whereas phorbol esters and IFN-γ both favour the development of monocytes.

IFN-γ inhibits the production of fully differentiated antibody-producing plasma cells from stimulated B-lymphocytes since this is dependent on cell division. In mice, IFN-γ is produced by T_{H1} helper cells which support the production of the IgG_{2a} subclass by polyclonally-activated B cells. IFN-γ is known to mediate this promotion of IgG_{2a} and to inhibit the IL-4-induced production of IgE. Thus, it may influence B-cell differentiation by influencing the nature of the B-cell isotype 'switch'.

INTERFERON-γ AND THE MAJOR HISTOCOMPATIBILITY COMPLEX

The surface of all nucleated cells contains integral membrane proteins coded by the Class I genes of the MHC (see Chapter 1). These proteins restrict the activity of $CD8^+$ T-lymphocytes, including those which are specifically cytotoxic for virus-infected cells. Class II proteins are found on a limited range of cells and they restrict the interaction between these cells and helper T-lymphocytes.

Class I and II induction

Class I induction. It has been known for more than a decade that Type I interferons are able to increase the cell surface expression of Class I antigens and the $β_2$-microglobulin which is always associated with them (Lindahl *et al.*, 1976). IFN-γ also increases Class I expression and has a higher specific activity than IFN-α/β. Increases can be detected within 1 h of incubating the cells with IFN-γ (Rosa *et al.*, 1986). Class I molecules consist of a single polypeptide chain encoded within the MHC, together with a $β_2$-microglobulin which is essential for its expression in the membrane, and which is encoded elsewhere in the genome. Thus, IFN increases the expression of the genes for both polypeptide chains, located on different chromosomes, in a coordinated fashion. The mechanism, however, is unknown.

Class I antigens are expressed on almost all nucleated cells with few exceptions. Occasionally, tumours arise which fail to express these antigens, and several have been grown in tissue culture to produce cell lines. In these, IFN-γ can induce mRNA synthesis with or without cell surface expression. Figure 9.5 shows the results of a typical experiment showing the results of Class I induction by IFN-γ on a human colon carcinoma cell line. Both type I and II IFNs can induce Class I expression on cells.

Class II induction. IFN-γ is the only type of IFN which can induce the synthesis and expression of Class II molecules. IFN-γ both increases the level of expression of Class II molecules in cells which normally have these membrane proteins, and can induce *de novo* expression in cells which do not do so. Class II molecules in man are coded by the HLA-D region which contains three subloci: DP, DQ and DR. Class II antigens coded by each separate sublocus are normally present on all cells which express Class II molecules albeit in differing amounts. Recent work with fibroblasts has suggested that IFN-γ may cause differential induction of the different subloci and that HLA DQ antigens are the least readily induced of the three. In addition, IFN-γ may have variable effects in inducing MHC antigens, even between cell lines of similar tissue origin, such as melanoma cells.

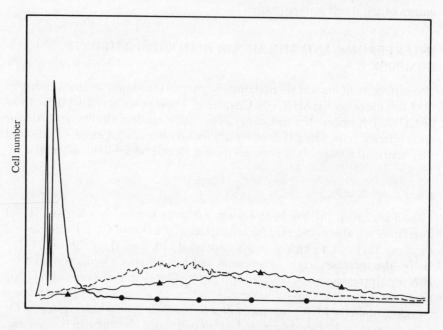

Fig. 9.5 Induction of MHC antigens by IFN-γ. The target cell is a human colon carcinoma line which was incubated with IFN-γ (1OU/ml) or IFN-γ+TNF-α for 3 days prior to incubation with an antibody to Class I determinants followed by fluorescein-conjugated anti-mouse immunoglobulin. The cells were analysed by cytofluorimetry. The graph shows the fluorescence intensity against cell number: ●——●, untreated; ———, IFN-γ; ▲——▲, IFN+TNF. The actual percentages of cells shown to be, separately, positive for Class I and for Class II (using another specific antibody) following several treatments are shown below:

Treatment	Class I	Class II
Untreated	15	1.8
IFN-γ	98	26
TNF-α (2OU/ml)	63	2.3
IFN-γ+TNF-α	98.5	56.8

(Graph and data courtesy of Diane Johnston, Paterson Research Institute)

Significance of IFN and MHC expression

Interferon which has been administered therapeutically in cancer has been found to increase the expression of MHC antigens on the patient's cells. So, for example, Class II antigens can be detected on epithelial and endothelial tissues which do not normally express these antigens. Similarly, in chronic inflammatory conditions such as rheumatoid arthritis where local immune responses cause the release of endogeneous IFN-γ, tissues in the vicinity are frequently found to express Class II molecules (Bottazzo *et al.*, 1986). Indeed, it is quite likely that such induction may be a normal, if (usually) localized and transient, feature of specific immune response which may promote immune responses in several ways:

Recognition of MHC antigens. Recognition of MHC antigens by lymphocytes is important in antigen presentation to helper T-cells and any increase in MHC antigens might be expected to promote this activity. The expression of Class I and II molecules by macrophages is sharply increased by recombinant IFN-γ but cocktails of lymphokines such as are found in the supernatants of activated lymphokines produce a much greater increase in the ability of these cells to present antigen (Isenberg *et al.*, 1986). In fact, the induction of MHC antigens *in vivo* is most likely to be the result of the release of several molecules from monocytes as well as lymphocytes. IL-4, TNF-α and TNF-β, for example, all induce MHC expression both separately and synergistically.

Recognition of Class I antigens. Recognition of Class I antigens is also essential for the specific destruction of virus-infected cells by cytotoxic T-lymphocytes (CTL). The induction of Class I molecules by interferons of all classes may result in more efficient destruction by these cells. Higher doses of IFN-α and IFN-β are required to induce Class I molecules but these may still be highly significant here since on release from an infected cell they may stimulate an increase of Class I molecules on that same cell and thus promote its destruction by CTL.

Class II antigens. The inappropriate expression of Class II molecules on tissues as a consequence of local release of endogenous IFN-γ by T-lymphocytes may trigger the start of some autoimmune reactions. Cells expressing Class II are typically antigen-presenting cells so that it is possible that these 'induced' cells may present 'self-antigen' to T-cells and thus trigger an 'anti-self' response (Bottazzo *et al.*, 1986). This response could become self-perpetuating since IFN-γ released as a result of the autoimmune reaction may trigger a further increase in Class II expression (Fig. 9.6). Several findings support this theory including the fact that thyroid cells taken from patients with autoimmune thyroiditis stain heavily with Class II antigens as do synovial cells obtained from the joints of patients with rheumatoid arthritis. Similarly, the localized sites of inflammation which occur in polymyositis and muscular dystrophy have been shown to be a source of IFN-γ and other lymphokines (Isenberg *et al.*, 1986). Tissue surrounding the inflammatory site binds the IFN-γ and this results in the expression of Class II molecules.

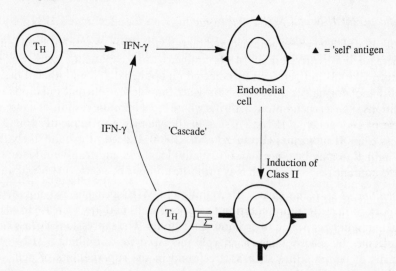

Fig. 9.6 IFN-γ and autoimmunity. Helper T-cells produce IFN-γ in response to specific antigen. Locally produced IFN-γ may induce Class II molecules on cells in the vicinity. These cells might then 'present' self-antigen to specific T-lymphocytes, setting up an autoimmune response and releasing further lymphokines.

NK cells. Tumour cell lines which are sensitive to NK cells are frequently devoid of some or all MHC antigens. However, the induction of MHC antigens on these cells by IFN-γ, is associated with a decrease in sensitivity to NK-mediated killing. These findings have led to speculation that the absence of MHC antigens may be related to recognition by NK cells.

INTERFERON-γ AND THE REGULATION OF OTHER CELL PROTEINS

IFN-γ increases the expression of several other membrane proteins in addition to MHC antigens. Amongst these is the β_2-microglobulin which is essential for the stable expression of Class I proteins but which is not encoded within the MHC itself (Heron *et al.*, 1978). IFN-γ also up-regulates expression of the CD4 molecule which is important in the function of helper T-lymphocytes but which also acts as the receptor for the human immunodeficiency virus, HIV. IFN-γ increases the level of cytoplasmic tubulin, the main protein of microtubules, which may be related to growth inhibition.

IFN-γ can greatly increase the expression, in myeloid cell lines as well as mature neutrophils and monocytes, of high-affinity receptors for the Fc region of IgG (FcγR) (Fridman *et al.*, 1980). These receptors are involved in enhancing the destruction of antibody-coated target cells by phagocytes and by large granular lymphocytes. An increase in the number of these receptors will increase the likelihood of antibody-coated cells interacting with the effector cell. IFN-γ is also known to down-regulate several proteins including cell surface transferrin receptors. The latter are abundant on actively dividing cells and are related to the increased uptake of iron by these cells. In this way, a reduction in the number of receptors may mediate some of the inhibition of proliferation mediated by interferon.

IFN-γ AND MACROPHAGES

In addition to their role as antigen-presenting cells for specific immune responses, monocytes and macrophages are important as non-specific effector cells. Their role extends from the phagocytosis of 'foreign' particles such as inhaled carbon (in tobacco smoke) and silica, to the ingestion and destruction of bacteria. Macrophages in particular form a major cellular defence against intracellular pathogens such as *Mycobacterium tuberculosis* and *Toxoplasma gondii*. Finally, macrophages have antitumour properties and can kill some tumour cell lines *in vitro*. The activity of macrophages is modified by the supernatants of mitogen-stimulated lymphocytes. These supernatants have, for some time, been known to contain a 'macrophage activation factor' (MAF) which has multiple effects on these cells (summarized in Table 9.3).

Macrophages destroy ingested bacteria either by the action of lysosomal enzymes or by the production of antimicrobial chemicals such as superoxide radicals. These latter are produced in the respiratory 'burst' which accompanies phagocytosis. A macrophage which has been activated by MAF is superior to the unstimulated form in phagocytic, bactericidal and tumoricidal capacity.

In recent years, it has become clear that the bulk of the MAF activity in the supernatants of activated lymphocytes can be attributed to IFN-γ (Nathan *et al.*, 1983; Svedersky *et al.*, 1984). The evidence that IFN-γ *is* MAF is extensive and includes the following.

(1) When macrophages are exposed *in vitro* to the conditioned medium from stimulated lymphocytes there is a burst of oxidative metabolism which increases the level of hydrogen peroxide several-fold. This increase can be completely abolished by the inclusion into the cultures of antibodies to IFN-γ.

Table 9.3 Properties of the activated macrophage

- Increases phagocytosis
- Increased cytotoxicity, e.g. to intracellular bacteria and tumour cells
- Increased cytostasis, e.g. to intracellular bacteria
- Increased motility
- More lysosomes
- Increased respiration and increased production of H_2O_2

---

(2)   Macrophages which have been treated with picomolar concentrations of IFN-γ ingest and kill bacteria, protozoal parasites and yeasts in far greater quantities than untreated cells. The lymphocytes of newborn babies produce very little IFN-γ in response to *in vitro* stimulation with concanavalin A (Wilson *et al.*, 1986) in contrast to the production of IL-2 which is similar to adult levels. This intrinsic, and transient, deficiency of IFN-γ may account for the great susceptibility of the human neonate to infection with intracellular pathogens.

(3)   Monocytes from cancer patients who have been treated with IFN-γ produce far more hydrogen peroxide than monocytes from untreated patients. The effect on the monocytes is rapid and can be detected as early as 60 min post-administration.

In addition to stimulating macrophages as effector cells, IFN-γ may also influence the ability of these cells to present antigen, since it increases the expression of Class II molecules of the MHC. Recognition of Class II molecules by helper T-cells is essential for the initiation of the lymphokine cascade and the greater the density of these molecules on the cell surface, the more likely it is that the helper T-cells will respond.

INTERFERON AND NATURAL KILLER (NK) CELLS

The antitumour effects of IFNs may to some extent be mediated by the stimulation of NK cells. NK cells show spontaneous cytotoxicity to some tumour lines (and virus-infected cells) *in vitro* although their precise function *in vivo* is uncertain (most cells from fresh tumours are resistant to NK killing). Interactions between NK cells and interferons occur on several levels and include the following:

- The cytotoxicity of NK cells is increased dramatically after incubation of these cells with IFNs of all classes.
- NK cells release IFN-α on contact with tumour target cells.
- NK cells are able to produce IFN-γ, the main stimulus for its release being IL-2 released in immune responses by helper T-cells (Trinchieri *et al.*, 1984).

Although NK cells rarely kill fresh tumour cells *in vitro*, it is possible that they may destroy small tumour foci as these arise in the body. Any tumours that become established may then be selected for NK resistance. The positive regulation of NK cytotoxicity by IFNs may be mediated by one or more mechanisms. First, IFN may hasten the maturation of an immature NK cell into one which is fully functional or IFN may increase the capacity of individual NK cells to recycle, i.e. to lyse several target cells in a sequential fashion. The ability of NK cells to recycle is suggested both by the kinetics of lysis *in vitro* and by the ratios of effector: target cells which are able to bring about lysis. IFN may serve to increase the rate at which NK cells recycle or to prolong the life of the recycling cell.

While the importance of the NK cell in immunity to tumours is uncertain, there is no doubt that these cells have a role *in vivo* in immune mechanisms against viral infections. For example, mice whose NK cells have been destroyed (by administration of antibodies directed against NK-specific membrane determinants) are very prone to a variety of viral infections, including herpes simplex and cytomegalovirus. The role of the NK cells in these situations is most likely to restrict the growth of the virus until such time as specific cytotoxic T-lymphocytes have been generated. Paradoxically, IFN treatment of an NK susceptible target cell frequently renders them less susceptible to NK-mediated lysis and this may be related in some way to the induction of MHC antigens on these cells (Trinchieri *et al.*, 1981).

IFN-γ AND ANTIBODY PRODUCTION

The effect of IFN-γ on antibody production depends primarily on the time of administration. For example, if given early on in an immune response, IFN-γ suppresses antibody production. This effect is a direct result of the inhibitory effects of IFN-γ on cell proliferation. However, when IFN-γ is administered late in an immune response, there may be increased antibody production. This increase reflects the ability of this interferon to enhance the differentiated functions of cells (in this case, secretion of immunoglobulin). Similar results are obtained whether measuring antibody production *in vivo* or *in vitro*. In mice, incubation of IFN-γ with polyclonally activated B-cells promotes the production of the IgG_{2a} subclass of antibody and suppresses the production of IgE and IgA (Finkelman *et al.*, 1988; O'Garra, 1988).

Thus it can be clearly seen that IFN-γ has potent immunomodulatory activities and can promote the activity of several cells involved in the production of an immune response. The immunomodulatory nature of this molecule has provided a rationale for testing IFN-γ in a variety of medical conditions, including cancer and viral illness. In addition, the involvement of this lymphokine in a number of pathological situations is currently under investigation.

IFN-γ and disease

There are now several clinical situations in which treatment with IFN-γ has potential or established benefits. IFN-γ has undergone clinical trials for the treatment of cancer and is potentially useful for the treatment of immune deficiency, including AIDS. Although IFN-γ has, by definition, antiviral activity, it is the classical IFNs (α and β) which are actually produced in response to viral infection. These latter have principally been used to treat viral infections, although it is to be expected that IFN-γ would produce similar results.

In addition to the use of IFN-γ as a therapeutic drug, this lymphokine may well be involved in the development of some pathologies, including autoimmune disease.

IFN-γ AND IMMUNODEFICIENCY

It now seems likely that all patients infected with the human immunodeficiency virus (AIDS) will eventually develop the AIDS-related complex (ARC) followed by full-blown AIDS. ARC is defined as a syndrome characterized by two or more symptoms of specific, chronic, unexplained conditions for three months or more. In addition there must be two or more abnormal laboratory findings such as raised immunoglobulin levels, HIV antibodies, or low lymphocyte levels (Bradbeer, 1986). The CD4$^+$ helper T-cell is the target of this lytic virus and it therefore follows that the underlying immunological deficit in AIDS and ARC patients is the absence or reduction in lymphokines released by these patients. One approach to AIDS immunotherapy has been to attempt to replace these lymphokines, a process which has been greatly facilitated by the availability of the recombinant molecules. Replacement therapy has been attempted using IL-2 and this is discussed in Chapter 5. Experiments have shown that the lymphocytes of patients with AIDS, but not ARC, are deficient in the production of IFN-γ as might be expected given that IL-2 promotes the sequential release of IFN-γ as well as other lymphokines (Vilcek *et al.*, 1985). Thus, treatment of AIDS patients with IFN-γ may prove to be beneficial in the control of opportunistic infection. In fact, a cocktail of lymphokines would most likely provide the best replacement therapy. In support of this idea is the finding that TNF-α and IFN-γ act synergistically *in vitro* to destroy HIV-infected cells and to reduce the level of transcription of virus-derived DNA in chronically infected cells (Wong *et al.*, 1988).

Some patients with primary immune deficiency syndromes (i.e. an immune defect which is not secondary to another disease) unrelated to infection with HIV also exhibit low levels of IFN-γ production. Such patients may also benefit from replacement therapy.

IFN-γ AND TUMOUR THERAPY

The effects of interferons on tumour cell growth have been recorded since the 1970s when Type I interferon was found to inhibit the growth of several animal tumours (Gresser and Bourali-Mauri, 1972). Since the tumours used were of viral origin, it was assumed that the growth inhibition was related to antiviral activity. Subsequent findings that interferon was able to inhibit the growth of chemically induced tumours as well as those with known viral aetiology, have led to the conclusion that the inhibition is a direct effect on the tumour cells themselves. Most of the early clinical trials of interferon in the treatment of cancer patients involved the use of IFN-α purified from lymphoblastoid cell lines or from leukocytes stimulated with virus. The painstaking purification of IFN from the supernatants of infected leukocytes was considerably improved by the production of a monoclonal antibody to IFN-α which enabled the protein to be purified by affinity chromatography. Later, the use of recombinant IFN-α and IFN-β enabled pure IFN to be given in relatively large quantities and without contaminating cytokines. The use of IFN-γ for the treatment of cancer was initiated some time after the classical IFNs and some clinical trials are still under way. Theoretically, IFN-γ should prove to be a more effective antitumour agent since it is more wide-ranging in its immunomodulatory properties. Unfortunately, much of the euphoria surrounding the use of IFNs for the treatment of cancer has proved to be unfounded and there are very few tumours in which regressions are consistently produced. However, one such malignancy is 'hairy cell leukaemia' where administration of IFN is now the treatment of choice (Quesada *et al.*, 1984). Hairy cell leukaemia, in the absence of IFN is inevitably fatal and the leukaemic cells are not susceptible to the usual chemotherapeutic drugs. This makes it all the more astonishing that IFN works so well. In fact, IFN may be acting, not as an inhibitor of cell proliferation, but as an inducer of differentiation in the leukaemic cells, which appear to be subject to a differentiation 'block'.

IFN-γ-RELATED TOXICITY

All IFNs have some toxicity *in vivo* and these include fever, malaise, headaches, fatigue and extreme weight loss attributable to loss of appetite coupled with vomiting (Nethersell and Sikora, 1985). At higher doses, IFNs may induce disturbance of the central nervous system, resulting in confusion, and slow-wave sleep. Impurities in preparations of native IFNs are likely to exacerbate these effects. In particular, IL-1, IL-6 and TNF-α and TNF-β may also induce fever and produce 'flu-like' symptoms.

Reference has already been made to the relationship between IFN-γ induction of MHC Class II antigens and the development of autoimmune disease. Inappropriate Class II expression has been found in several autoimmune diseases including rheumatoid arthritis and may result in a self-perpetuating reaction against 'self' antigens presented by these Class II-positive cells (Klareskog *et al.*, 1982). In support of this idea is the finding that the more widespread use of IFN-γ for the treatment of cancer has been accompanied by an increase in autoimmune phenomena in these patients.

Molecular biology

Human IFN-γ is encoded by a single gene located on chromosome 12. Human IFN-α and IFN-β are encoded by genes on chromosome 9. Multiple genes encode at least 13 subtypes of IFN-α and two subtypes of IFN-β (Dijkman and Billiau, 1985). The subtypes of IFN-α differ in tissue specificity. IFN-α and IFN-β show a high degree of structural similarity with an amino acid homology of approximately 29%. Thus they appear to have evolved from a common ancestral gene, the genes having diverged an estimated 500 million years ago. There is very

Table 9.4   Comparison of human IFNs α, β and γ and their genes

Property	IFN-α	IFN-β	IFN-γ
Chromosomal location of gene in humans	9	9	12
Number of subtypes	13	2	1
Introns in gene?	No	No	3
Chromosomal location of human IFN receptor gene	21	21	6
Amino acid residues in secreted molecule	165/6	166	146
Length of signal polypeptide	23	21	20
Glycosylation of IFN?	No	1 site	2 sites
Stability of IFN at pH 2	Stable	Stable	Labile
Stability at 56°C	Stable	Stable	Labile

little, if any, structural homology between IFN-α and IFN-β, and IFN-γ. A comparison of the properties of these three interferons and their genes is shown in Table 9.4.

Human IFN-γ is now available in a pure form as a result of recombinant DNA technology and has been cloned in both prokaryotes such as *E. coli* and eukaryotes such as Chinese hamster ovary (CHO) and yeast cells. Mature IFN-γ is a protein of 146 amino acids (17 kDa) with an excess of basic amino acid residues. The protein, which is both heat and acid labile, is differentially N-glycosylated to yield two forms with molecular weights of 20 K and 25 K, respectively. Like most glycosylated lymphokines, the significance of glycosylation is not fully understood although it is known that unglycosylated IFN-γ is preferentially taken up into the liver. Recombinant, prokaryotic IFN-γ has the same specific activity as the native form.

MECHANISM OF ACTION

All interferons mediate their effects following interaction with a specific cell surface receptor. IFN-γ uses a specific receptor encoded by a gene on chromosome 6 in humans and which is not used by any other interferon class (Rashidbargi *et al.*, 1986). In contrast IFN-α and IFN-β share a common receptor encoded by a gene located on chromosome 21. The density of IFN-γ receptors has been estimated by radiolabelled binding assays at approximately 10 000 per single HeLa cell and 2400 per human fibroblast. The high-affinity binding ($K_d = 3.3 \times 10^{-10}$ M) is characteristic of many hormone-like receptor–ligand interactions. Individual cells express receptors of one affinity only, in contrast with IL-1 and IL-2 where high- and low-affinity receptors are seen. However, two different molecular forms of the IFN-γ receptor have been found on different cells: those on HeLa cells having a molecular weight of 120 kDa when bound to IFN-γ, and those on monocytes banding on

SDS–PAGE at 165 kDa. In fact, the receptor found on monocytes may be unique to cells of that lineage and its presence may be related to the activity of IFN-γ in producing 'activation' of these cells (Orchansky *et al.*, 1986). All human cells have receptors for IFN-γ and this ubiquity probably relates to its antiviral, rather than immunomodulatory, activity.

Although a large number of receptors may be present, there is no need for saturation of these receptors to stimulate biological activity. In fact, the number of receptors which have to be filled depends on the activity which is being measured (Rubinstein *et al.*, 1987). For example, the induction of MHC antigens requires only an estimated 40–60 molecules of bound IFN-γ to achieve maximum activity whereas IFN-γ-induced resistance to NK cytotoxicity needs much higher numbers. There are some indications that the different functions of this IFN-γ may be mediated by different parts of the molecule. Monoclonal antibodies, prepared against different epitopes on the murine IFN-γ molecule, were found to have differential effects on macrophage activation with antibodies either enhancing or inhibiting macrophage activity. On the other hand, all antibodies were shown to inhibit antiviral activity.

Summary

Interferon-γ is a lymphokine with potent immunomodulatory activities in addition to its antiviral role. Some of these properties are found in classical interferons although IFN-γ often exhibits a higher specific activity. In addition, IFN-γ is unique amongst the interferons in activating macrophages and in the induction of Class II molecules of the MHC. The activation of macrophages is important in the killing of intracellular parasites and possibly tumour cells *in vivo*. The induction of Class II molecules may facilitate antigen presentation to helper T-cells, although inappropriate expression may be implicated in the development of autoimmune disease. IFN-γ has therapeutic value in the treatment of a very limited range of tumours and may prove to be useful as part of a drug 'cocktail' for immune replacement in AIDS or AIDS-related complex.

References

Andersson, U., Laskay, T., Andersson, J., Kiessling, R. and DeLey, M. (1986). 'Phenotypic characterisation of individual IFN-γ producing cells after OKT3 antibody activation', *Eur. J. Immunol.* **16**, p. 1457.

Ball, E. D., Guyre, P. M., Shen, L. *et al.* (1984). 'IFN-γ induces monocytoid differentiation in the HL60 cell line', *J. Clin. Invest.* **73**, p. 1072.

Beresini, M. H., Lempert, M. J. and Epstein, L. B. (1988). 'Overlapping polypeptide induction in human fibroblasts in response to treatment with IFN-α, IFN-γ, IL-1α, IL-1β and TNF', *J. Immunol.* **140**, p. 485.

Billiau, A. (1987). 'Interferon β_2 as a promoter of growth and differentiation of B cells', *Immunol. Today* **8**, p. 84.

Bottazzo, G. F., Pujol-Barrell, R., Hanafusa, T. and Feldman, M. (1986). 'Organ-specific autoimmunity: a 1986 overview', *Immunol. Rev.* **94**, p. 137.

Bradbeer, C. (1986). 'AIDS – epidemiology and screening', *Med. Inter.* **2**, p. 1241.

Czarniecki, C. W., Fennie, C., Powers, D. B. and Estell, D. A. (1984). 'Synergistic antiviral and antiproliferative activities of *Escherichia coli* derived human alpha, beta and gamma interferons', *J. Virol.* **49**, p. 490.

Dijkman, R. and Billiau, A. (1985). 'An introduction to the genes of the interferon system' in *Interferons: Their Impact in Biology and Medicine*, ed. Taylor-Papadimitriou, J. Oxford, Oxford University Press Medical Publications.

Finkelman, F. D., Katona, I. M., Mosmann, T. R. and Coffman, R. L. (1988). 'Interferon-γ regulates the isotypes of immunoglobulin secreted during *in vivo* humoral immune responses', *J. Immunol.* **140**, p. 1022.

Fridman, W. H., Gresser, I., Bandu, M. T. *et al.* (1980). 'Interferon enhances the expression of Fcγ receptors', *J. Immunol.* **124**, p. 2436.

Gresser, I. and Bourali-Maury, C. (1970). 'Antitumour effects of interferon preparations in mice', *J. Natl Cancer Inst.* **45**, p. 365.

Gresser, I. and Bourali-Maury, C. (1972). 'Inhibition by interferon preparations of a solid malignant tumour and pulmonary metastasis in mice', *Nature (New Biol.)* **236**, p. 78.

Heron, I., Hokland, M. and Berg, K. (1978). 'Enhanced expression of β2M and HLA antigens, on human lymphoid cells by interferon', *Proc. Natl Acad. Sci. (USA)* **75**, p. 6215.

Isaacs, A. and Lindenmann, J. (1957). 'Virus interference. I. Interferons', *Proc. Roy. Soc. (London)* **147**, p. 258.

Isenberg, D. A., Rowe, D., Shearer, M. *et al.* (1986). 'Localisation of interferons and IL-2 in polymyositis and muscular dystrophy', *Clin. Exp. Immunol.* **63**, p. 450.

Kasahara, T., Hooks, J. J., Doughterty, S. F. and Oppenheim, J. J. (1983). 'IL-2 mediated immune interferon (IFN-γ) production by human T cells and T cell subsets', *J. Immunol.* **130**, p. 1784.

Klareskog, L., Forsum, U., Scheynius, A. *et al.* (1982). 'Evidence in support of a self-perpetuating HLA-DR-dependent delayed-type cell reaction in rheumatoid arthritis', *Proc. Natl Acad. Sci. (USA)* **79**, p. 3632.

Kronke, M., Leonard, W. J., Depper, J. M. and Greene, W. C. (1985). 'Sequential expression of genes involved in human T lymphocyte growth and differentiation', *J. Exp. Med.* **161**, p. 1593.

Lindahl, P., Gresser, I., Leary, P. and Tovey, M. (1976). 'IFN treatment of mice: enhanced expression of histocompatibility antigens on lymphoid cells', *Proc. Natl Acad. Sci. (USA)* **73**, p. 1284.

Nathan, C. F., Murray, H. W., Wiebe, M. E. and Rubin, B. Y. (1983). 'Identification of IFN-γ as the lymphokine that activates human macrophage oxidative metabolism and antimicrobial activity', *J. Exp. Med.* **158**, p. 670.

Nethersell, A. and Sikora, K. (1985). 'Interferons and malignant disease' in *Interferons: Their Impact in Biology and Medicine*, Ed. Taylor-Papadimitriou, J. Oxford, Oxford University Press Medical Publications.

O'Garra, A. (1988). 'The pleiotropic effects of B cell growth factor, *Immunol. Today* **8**, p. 44.

Orchansky, P., Rubinstein, M. and Fischer, D. G. (1986). The interferon-γ receptor in human monocytes is different from the one in non-hematopoietic cell', *J. Immunol.* **136**, p. 169.

Quesada, J. R., Reuben, J., Manning, J. T. *et al.* (1984). 'Alpha-interferon for the induction of remission in hairy cell leukaemia' *New Engl. J. Med.* **310**, p. 15.

Rashidbargi, A., Langer, J. A., Jung, V. *et al.* (1986). The gene for the human immune interferon receptor is located on chromosome 6. *Proc. Natl Acad. Sci. (USA)* **83**, p. 384.

Rosa, F. M., Cochet, M. M. and Fellous, M. (1986). 'Interferon and major histocompatibility complex genes: a model to analyse eukaryotic gene regulation', in *Interferon* **7**; p. 47. London, Academic Press.

Rubin, B. Y. and Gupta, S. L. (1980). 'Differential efficacies of human Type I and Type II interferons as anti-viral and anti-proliferative agents', *Proc. Natl Acad. Sci. (USA)* **77**, p. 5928.

Rubinstein, M., Novick, D. and Fischer, D. G. (1987). 'The human interferon-γ receptor system', *Immunol. Rev.* **97**, p. 29.

Sandvig, S., Laskay, T., Andersson, J., DeLey, M. and Andersson, U. (1987). 'Gamma-interferon is produced by CD3$^+$ and CD3$^-$ lymphocytes', *Immunol. Rev.* **97**, p. 51.

Stewart, W. E., Blalock, J. E., Burke, D. C. *et al.* (1980). 'Interferon nomenclature', *J. Immunol.* **125**, p. 2353.

Svedersky, L. P., Benton, C. V., Berger, W. H. *et al.* (1984). 'Biological and antigenic similarities of murine interferon and macrophage activation factor', *J. Exp. Med.* **159**, p. 812.

Trinchieri, G., Granato, D. and Perussia, B. (1981). 'IFN-induced resistance of fibroblasts to cytolysis mediated by NK cells: specificity and mechanism,' *J. Immunol.* **126**, p. 335.

Trinchieri, G., Matsumoto-Kobayashi, M., Clark, S. C. *et al.* (1984). 'Response of resting human peripheral blood NK cells to IL-2', *J. Exp. Med.* **160**, p. 1147.

Van Wauwe, J. P., De Mey, J. R. and Goosens, J. G. (1980). 'OKT3: a monoclonal anti-human T lymphocyte antibody with potent mitogenic properties', *J. Immunol.* **124**, p. 2708.

Vilcek, J., Henrikson-Destefano, D., Siegal, D. *et al.* (1985). 'Regulation of IFN-γ induction in human peripheral blood cells by exogenous and endogenously produced IL-2', *J. Immunol.* **135**, p. 1851.

Wheelock, E. F. (1965). 'Interferon-like virus-inhibitor induced in human leukocytes by phytohaemagglutinin', *Science* **149**, p. 310.

Wilson, C. B., Westall, J., Johnston, L. *et al.* (1986). 'Decreased production of IFN-γ by human neonatal cells. Intrinsic and regulatory deficiencies', *Eur. J. Immunol.* **77**, p. 860.

Wong, G. H. W., Krowka, J. F., Stites, D. P. and Greddel, D. V. (1988). '*In vitro* anti-HIV activities of TNF-α and IFN-γ', *J. Immunol.* **140**, p. 120.

10

Tumour Necrosis Factor

Introduction

The supernatants of endotoxin-treated macrophages produce a protein which can destroy tumour tissue in a tumour-bearing animal. This protein, known as 'tumour necrosis factor' (TNF) was discovered during investigations of the host–tumour response. Tumour immunology is a discipline which began with the premise that malignant tumours can provoke an immune response in the animal in which they arise. Such a premise is based on the assumption that tumours have 'foreign' antigenic determinants which induce immune responses against the tumour. Tumour immunology therefore investigates the following:

- The extent to which tumour-bearing individuals mount immune responses towards their tumour
- The cells and macromolecules involved in the immune response towards tumours (if any)
- The ways in which antitumour responses can be manipulated with a view to controlling the tumour by immunotherapy

Animal models have been used extensively in tumour immunology, and one such system which has been thoroughly studied is the carcinogen-induced transplantable tumour system in rodents, illustrated in Fig. 10.1. Powerful carcinogens such as 3-methylcholanthrene readily induce primary tumours in laboratory animals and these tumours can be maintained by transplanting them to syngeneic (i.e. genetically identical) animals. If the tumours are transplanted subcutaneously, their growth can be easily monitored under different conditions. This system was used extensively, and successfully, to demonstrate that animals can, and do, make effective cell-mediated immune response to carcinogen-induced tumours (Baldwin *et al.*, 1973). Humoral immune responses are also seen but rarely does tumour-specific antibody cause destruction of the tumour. However,

3-MCA

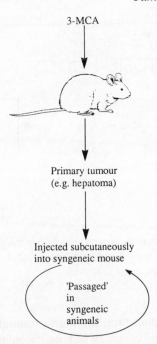

Primary tumour
(e.g. hepatoma)

Injected subcutaneously
into syngeneic mouse

'Passaged'
in
syngeneic
animals

Fig. 10.1 Transplantable tumours. The primary tumour is induced in mice or rats using a carcinogen such as 3-methylcholanthrene (3-MCA). The tumour is excised and can be transplanted to syngeneic (from the same highly inbred strain) animals, where it will not be rejected as a transplant. Small pieces of the tumour are transplanted in a subcutaneous position so that growth, and the effects of different treatments, can be readily monitored.

when human tumour immunity was investigated, it was somewhat disappointing to discover that human tumours rarely evoke such powerful responses as carcinogen-induced tumours in animals.

Enthusiasm for tumour immunology was rekindled by the discovery that several naturally occurring substances with immunomodulatory properties could stimulate antitumour effects in cancer patients as well as experimental animals. One of the earliest of the 'biological response modifiers' used to treat cancer patients was Bacillus Calmette-Guérin (BCG) an attenuated strain of *Mycobacterium bovis* which is most commonly used to immunize against tuberculosis. Mycobacteria are potent activators of monocytes and macrophages, which, after stimulation, frequently display tumoricidal activity. For this reason, BCG was extensively tested for its anticancer properties, and particularly against several kinds of leukaemia. Extensive clinical trials with BCG have, however, proved disappointing, in that tumour regressions could neither be induced nor maintained.

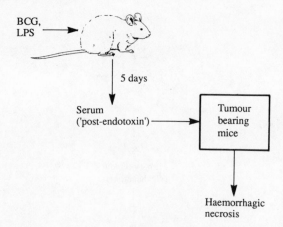

Fig. 10.2 Haemorrhagic necrosis. Several days after mice have been treated with endotoxin (LPS) and BCG, their serum contains a factor which causes haemorrhagic necrosis of established tumours in other mice.

In 1975, carcinogen-induced transplantable tumours in animals were used to demonstrate that the serum of mice which had been injected several days earlier with BCG and endotoxin could cause 'haemorrhagic necrosis' of transplantable tumours when injected into tumour-bearing animals (Fig. 10.2) (Carswell *et al.*, 1975). Haemorrhagic necrosis of tumours is characterized by bleeding from blood vessels within the tumour itself. Under such conditions, the tumour blackens and eventually dries up to form a scab. Necrosis could be induced by 'tumour necrosis serum' but not by endotoxin alone, indicating an indirect effect of the endotoxin on host cells. It was therefore suggested that endotoxin stimulates the production of a 'tumour necrosis factor' (TNF) which caused haemorrhagic necrosis when transferred to a tumour-bearing animal.

COLEY'S TOXINS

The history of TNF is a splendid illustration of recent scientific discoveries being able to explain the medical treatments which had been adopted empirically by clinicians several decades earlier. Immunological interest in post-endotoxin serum can be traced back to observations, made almost a century ago by Sir William Coley which resulted in the use of 'Coley's toxins' in the treatment of cancer. Coley's toxins were preparations of killed bacteria which were administered to cancer patients to stimulate regression of a tumour. This treatment was based on observations that tumours sometimes diminished, or occasionally regressed altogether, in patients who were undergoing an active bacterial infection. The use of Coley's toxins formed the basis for post-surgical cancer therapy a century ago but their use died out with the availability of powerful chemotherapeutic agents and the refinement of the techniques of radiotherapy. With hindsight, it seems likely that some at least of the effects of Coley's toxins can be attributed to the induction of TNF in the cancer patient (Old, 1988).

TUMOUR NECROSIS FACTOR AND LYMPHOTOXIN

Tumour necrosis factor, induced in endotoxin-treated animals, is produced by monocytes and macrophages which have phagocytosed the bacterial product. Its relationship to a molecule with similar properties, produced by lymphocytes, has only in the last few years been clarified. Over 20 years ago, the supernatants of antigen-stimulated lymphocytes were found to contain a factor which could kill syngeneic lymphocytes *in vitro*. This factor, called lymphotoxin (LT), was released 24 h after incubation of sensitized cells with the specific antigen (Ruddle and Waksman, 1967). Functionally, the activities of TNF and lymphotoxin are indistinguishable and recent cloning of the genes for both molecules has revealed a high degree of homology. Other similarities, including gene location and organization, and the fact that the two molecules compete for the same cell surface receptor on target cells, have led to a proposed nomenclature in which the original macrophage-derived TNF becomes TNF-α and lymphotoxin becomes TNF-β, a terminology which will be adopted in this chapter.

Activities of TNF

'Tumour necrosis factor' is a somewhat misleading term, emphasizing as it does only a single facet of the activities of these molecules. In fact, TNF has many other biological effects, some of which are listed in Table 10.1. TNF is a true interleukin according to the 'official' definition although it has no IL number assigned to it. The range of activities supported by this molecule is reminiscent of

Table 10.1 Activities of TNF

- Haemorrhagic necrosis of tumours *in vivo*
- Cytostatic and cytotoxic effects on tumour cells *in vitro*
- Activation of polymorphonuclear leukocytes
- Increasing adhesiveness of endothelial cells
- Up-regulation of MHC antigens
- Stimulation of IL-1 release
- Delayed hypersensitivity reactions
- Acute phase inflammatory reactions: acute phase proteins and fever
- Stimulation of collagenase
- Stimulate osteoclast activity
- Increase prostaglandin synthesis

IL-1 and indeed the two molecules share many similar properties (though unrelated structurally). TNF also synergizes with IFN, for example, in inhibiting the growth of cultured tumour cells, or inducing the expression of MHC antigens.

TNF can have both beneficial and harmful effects *in vivo*. For example, it is a powerful inflammatory agent both in its own right and also because it stimulates the production of IL-1 by macrophages. However, as a result of its inflammatory nature, TNF is also implicated in a number of disease processes including septic shock, an acute and sometimes fatal syndrome accompanying some bacterial infections. Moreover, chronic production of TNF as a consequence of long-term bacterial or parasitic infection can result in permanent tissue damage including excessive loss of weight and 'wasting' of muscles. TNF is also implicated in the chronic inflammatory reactions of certain autoimmune diseases such as auto-immune thyroiditis and Type I (insulin-dependent) diabetes.

Clinically, TNF holds some promise as an antitumour agent especially when combined with interferon. On the other hand, if TNF causes or exacerbates certain diseases, then treatment with TNF inhibitors (monoclonal antibodies for example) may provide a useful therapy.

TNF AND TUMOURS

Undoubtedly much interest in TNF has been generated as a consequence of its tumoricidal properties. The action of TNF on tumours is not species-specific, so that murine TNF is able to cause necrosis of human tumours which have been transplanted into athymic mice (to prevent them being rejected as a transplant). Although the precise mechanism of the induction of haemorrhagic necrosis is unknown, the action of TNF can, at least in part, be attributed to its inflammatory properties, which are discussed below.

In addition to causing haemorrhagic necrosis *in vivo*, both TNF-α and TNF-β kill, or inhibit the growth of, malignant cells *in vitro* and again, this activity is not species-specific. A combination of IFN-γ and TNF has proven to be more lethal than either of these lymphokines alone but the mechanism of this synergy is uncertain (Feinman *et al.*, 1987). Interleukin-1 is also directly tumoricidal *in vitro* and a combination of TNF and IL-1 can have additive or synergistic effects.

The implication from these experiments is that TNF, possibly in combination with other proteins, may also have a direct cytotoxic effect on tumours *in vivo* and, if so, this gives further encouragement for testing its activity in cancer patients. The mechanism of TNF-induced haemorrhagic necrosis is still uncertain but the destruction of the tumour is partly the indirect result of the action of TNF on the endothelial cells lining the walls of tumour-associated blood vessels. Direct and indirect cytotoxicity do not always go hand-in-hand and some tumours which are destroyed by TNF *in vivo*, are not sensitive to its activity *in vitro*. A good example of this is the 'Meth A' sarcoma, a transplantable murine tumour which provided the animal model with which TNF was discovered originally. These tumour cells, though effectively destroyed by haemorrhagic necrosis, are not killed by direct action *in vitro*. It seems likely therefore that the inflammatory effects of TNF, attracting PMNs and promoting bleeding in tumour-associated blood vessels, are very important in these cases. In addition, other cytokines are available *in vivo* which can synergize with TNF in the destruction of tumour cells.

Direct toxicity

Cell lines derived from a range of malignant tumours show differential susceptibilities to TNF-induced killing and this does not always correlate with the number of receptors on a susceptible line. The actual mechanism of tumour cell destruction mediated by TNF is unclear although several hypotheses have been proposed. These suggestions include:

(1) *Fragmentation of DNA*. This is seen in several cultures following treatment with TNF. Fragmentation could be the result of a TNF-induced alteration in the permeability of the nuclear membrane which allows a cytoplasmic DNAse to enter the nucleus (Ruddle, 1985).

(2) *Induction of free radicals*. TNF treatment of cells induces the synthesis of prostaglandins from phospholipid-derived arachidonic acid in the membrane. Highly toxic free radicals, capable of acting at multiple sites in the cell, are generated via this pathway. In support of this theory, it is known that drugs such as aspirin, which interfere with the synthesis of prostaglandins, also reduce TNF toxicity (Matthews *et al.*, 1987).

(3) *Uncontrolled hydrolysis of ATP*. Treatment of muscle cells with TNF causes hydrolysis of ATP with energy being released as heat (Ruddle, 1987). A cycle may be set up in which uncontrolled ATP hydrolysis drains the energy reserves in the cell, leading to excess lactate production, lowering pH, causing more hydrolysis of ATP, etc. This futile cycle, which leads to excess heat, can destroy the cell.

(4) *Induction of cellular proteases*. The induction of proteases and the activation of lysosomal enzymes may result in cellular autolysis. Proteases have for some time been implicated in the direct cell–cell killing by cytotoxic T-lymphocytes and natural killer cells.

TNF AND INFLAMMATION

Administration of TNF to animals causes an acute phase response which in many ways is similar to that induced by IL-1, i.e. fever, synthesis of acute phase proteins and increases in the amino acids and neutrophil content in the blood. While TNF can mediate some of these effects by direct interaction with the target cells, the majority are attributable to the synthesis of IL-1 by endothelial cells and macrophages which is induced by TNF. The injection of recombinant TNF into experimental animals, however, causes a biphasic fever, indicating that both

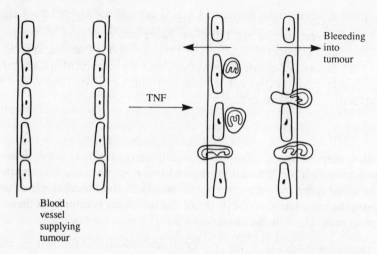

Fig. 10.3   TNF and inflammation. When TNF is injected into tumour-bearing animals, the blood vessels supplying the tumour become inflamed. There is an increase in an adhesion molecule which causes more neutrophils to adhere to these vessels and to move across the basement membrane through gaps between the endothelial cells. In addition, bleeding occurs across these vessels, resulting in swelling and blackening of the tumour.

TNF and the induced IL-1 can act on the temperature regulatory centre in the hypothalamus (Dinarello *et al.*, 1986).

Haemorrhagic necrosis of tumours may also be related to the inflammatory effect of TNF on the endothelial cells of blood vessels (Fig. 10.3) which leads to an accumulation of neutrophils in tumours, as well as some uninvolved organs. During inflammation, endothelial cells move apart, and neutrophils adhere to them via adhesion molecules on their membranes. The neutrophils then move across the vessel wall between the endothelial cells. TNF influences the number of neutrophils which emerge from blood vessels into tissues by increasing the expression of the neutrophil adhesion molecules so that more cells move across (Gamble *et al.*, 1985). In addition TNF also causes 'preferential' bleeding in tumour-associated blood vessels and a few normal tissues, and this may be related to an alteration of the properties of the endothelial cells lining the blood vessels.

TNF AND THE INDUCTION OF MHC ANTIGENS

TNF may alter immune responses by modulating the expression of MHC glycoproteins which are closely involved in T-cell recognition of foreign antigens. The possible immunological 'benefits' of increased MHC expression have previously been described in other chapters and include (i) more efficient antigen presentation resulting from increased Class II expression, and (ii) more efficient cytolysis of virus-infected cells resulting from increased Class I expression. TNF increases the level of expression of both Class I and Class II antigens on cells which normally express them (Scheurich *et al.*, 1986) and can even promote *de novo* expression of Class II on non-expressing cells. Synergisms between TNF and IFN-γ are also seen. Like IFN-γ, TNF has also been implicated in the development of autoimmune disease by stimulating endothelial cells to present 'self' antigens together with induced Class II antigens, to T-lymphocytes. In addition, TNF induces the synthesis of IL-1 by endothelial cells so that these cells could themselves supply all the signals necessary to stimulate a T-lymphocyte.

Evidence implicating TNF in autoimmune disease has come from a study of Type I diabetes, an autoimmune disease in which there is destruction of the insulin-producing β-cells of the islets of Langerhans. Islet cells in pancreatic biopsies of patients are found to express Class II molecules whereas 'normal' islet cells can only be induced to express Class II by incubation with a combination of IFN-γ and TNF (Pujol-Barrell *et al.*, 1987).

TNF AND PARASITE INFECTION

The precise role of TNF *in vivo* has yet to be elucidated definitively. There are, however, good reasons to believe that it plays an important role in the immune response against parasites (Wozebcraift *et al.*, 1984). The evidence for this suggestion includes the following findings:

(1) When mice have been injected with TNF, they are found to be more resistant to some forms of malaria. In addition, TNF may alter the course of the disease and render a fatal form, non-fatal.
(2) TNF increases the cytotoxicity of eosinophils towards the larvae of various parasites including schistosomes.
(3) Increased levels of TNF can be detected in the serum of patients with parasitic infections.

However, the role of TNF in anti-parasite immunity is controversial since, in mice where malaria has entered the brain, antibodies to TNF inhibit a TNF-induced inflammation in brain cells which would otherwise prove fatal (Grau *et al.*, 1987).

TNF AND CACHEXIA

Cachexia is the profound loss of weight and wasting of muscle which sometimes occurs in patients with chronic bacterial infection or parasitic infestation. This condition is also seen in animals with parasitic worms and is therefore of economic and clinical significance, especially in Third World countries. Cattle with an apparently trivial parasitic burden can suffer as much as a 50% loss of weight and, similarly, individuals who are malnourished already may have their lives threatened by an extreme weight loss. Cachexia is also seen in cancer patients, often before their condition has been diagnosed.

Cachectin is a molecule which was first isolated from the culture supernatants of endotoxin-treated mouse macrophages, which caused cachexia when injected into normal mice (Cerami and Beutler, 1988). Extensive biochemical analysis of this molecule has revealed its identity as TNF-α.

Cachexia occurs as the result of several TNF-induced activities, including the following:

Inhibition of lipoprotein lipase (LPL)

This is an enzyme found in adipose tissue which is essential for the normal storage of fat. In cachectic individuals, the activity of LPL is greatly reduced and this results in the loss of stored fat. LPL has been studied in cultured adipocytes and the addition of serum from endotoxin-treated mice to these cells results in a loss of LPL activity. Similarly, supernatants from macrophages treated with endotoxin are also inhibitory. It seems likely that TNF acts directly on LPL to inhibit its activity. On the other hand, both IL-1 and IFN can contribute to cachexia by inhibiting the activity of LPL (Beutler *et al.*, 1985).

Proteolysis of muscle

TNF induces the synthesis of IL-1, which stimulates proteolysis of muscle, and therefore increases the levels of amino acids in the plasma (Nawroth *et al.*, 1986).

Mobilization of amino acids provides the building blocks for the synthesis of macromolecules such as the acute phase proteins, and is beneficial, at least in the short term. Fats may also be necessary to provide the energy to drive the synthetic and proliferative activities which take place during an immune response. Clearly, though, drastic weight losses, if unchecked, can be positively harmful to an individual whose health is otherwise undermined by a large tumour, by parasites or by general undernourishment. The problem of weight loss is exacerbated by the effect of TNF (possibly through IL-1) in suppressing appetite. Identification of the molecule(s) responsible for cachexia provides a means by which cachexia can be limited by, for example, administration of monoclonal antibodies to TNF. One problem which needs also to be addressed is the nature of the tumour-associated and parasite-associated molecules which stimulate TNF production in the first place. Finding the nature of the stimulating molecule might again provide a handle for preventing cachexia. In bacterial infection, the stimulating molecule, lipopolysaccharide, is well known.

SEPTIC SHOCK

If animals are given too much bacterial endotoxin, death can occur as the result of endotoxic or septic shock. The symptoms of endotoxic shock (Table 10.2) are

Table 10.2 Symptoms of endotoxic shock

- Hypotension
- Diarrhoea
- Piloerection
- Metabolic acidosis
- Accumulation of neutrophils in lungs
- Haemorrhagic necrosis in pancreas and adrenals
- Necrosis in kidney

dramatic and occur rapidly after endotoxin treatment. Although the symptoms vary within different species, hypotension, diarrhoea and death from respiratory arrest can occur within hours of endotoxin treatment. Similar syndromes may occur as a result of a severe bacterial infection in which bacteria are found in the blood (bacteraemia). Septic shock can result from exotoxins as well as endotoxins and one which is becoming more prevalent is the 'toxic shock' syndrome (TSS). TSS occurs in young women using tampons contaminated with *Staphylococcus aureus*, and is associated with the bacterial exotoxin, TSST-1. Many of the symptoms of TSS may be attributable to TNF. Several pieces of evidence, discussed below, have shown that TNF is involved in the induction of septic shock (Tracey and Cerami, 1988):

(1) Mice injected with recombinant TNF which is free of contaminating endotoxin develop septic shock along with a profound accumulation of neutrophils into the lungs. These neutrophils may degranulate, losing lysosomal enzymes to the surrounding tissues, causing damage. The neutrophils accumulating in the lungs are highly phagocytic and bactericidal.
(2) Doses of endotoxin capable of inducing septic shock have been shown to result in the release of large amounts (in some cases as much as milligrams) of TNF from macrophages.
(3) Mice injected with antibodies to TNF can tolerate relatively high numbers of bacteria in the blood, without developing shock.
(4) Amongst a large number of humans admitted to hospital with septicaemia or meningococcal disease, there was a very strong correlation between detectable levels of TNF in the blood, and a fatal outcome of the disease. This may provide a rationale for the administration of anti-TNF antibodies to such patients (Waage *et al.*, 1987).

TNF-β AND AIDS

The human immunodeficiency virus (HIV) replicates within helper T-cells and destroys them by a mechanism which is as yet undefined. In patients who are infected with HIV leading to AIDS, there is a drastic reduction in the level of helper T-lymphocytes. The loss of T_H is due in part to destruction of the virus-infected cells by specific cytotoxic T-lymphocytes, which is the usual cell-mediated mechanism for eliminating viruses. However, in addition to specific CTL, there seems to be a lytic molecule produced within the infected cell which may also cause lysis. It has been suggested that the cytolytic molecule is TNF-β.

HIV possesses a trans-activating (*tat*) gene, which stimulates replication of the virus by activating the host's DNA. In doing so, HIV may also activate the host gene for TNF-β. The large amounts of TNF-β produced and released would be toxic, not only for the producer cell, but also for others with which it can become attached via the CD4 molecules (Fig. 10.4). If this does indeed occur, then

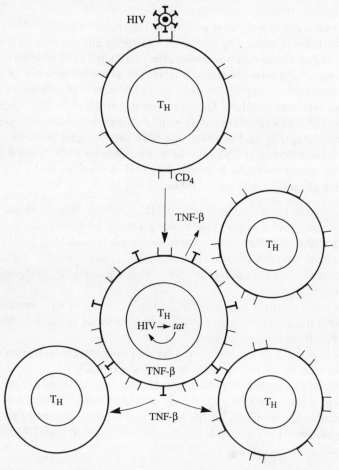

Fig. 10.4   HIV and lymphotoxin (TNF-β). HIV enters T-helper cells via the CD4 glycoprotein. The infected cell expresses viral protein and can therefore bind to other T_H via their own CD4. The result is a large clump of helper T-cells. The original infected cell produces TNF-β, possibly stimulated by the *tat* gene of HIV. The TNF-β may be responsible for lysis of the infected cell as well as those which are 'clumped' together.

antibodies to TNF-β would be expected to prevent the autolysis of helper T-lymphocytes and so prevent the loss of this important cell (Ruddle, 1986).

Cachexia is also prevalent in AIDS patients and in parts of Africa the disease has the colloquial name of 'slim disease' and this may also be related to TNF-β production by helper T-cells infected with the virus.

Production of TNF

A list of different sources of TNF is given in Table 10.3. TNF-α can be obtained from endotoxin-treated macrophage cell lines. TNF-β can be obtained from lectin-stimulated T-lymphocytes although this is contaminated with multiple lymphokines. Both helper and cytotoxic T-lymphocytes are capable of producing TNF-β when stimulated with antigen in the presence of accessory cells such as macrophages. Alternatively, some T-cell hybridomas secrete TNF-β constitutively, without this requirement. Both TNF-α and TNF-β can be produced by several cell lines *in vitro*. RPMI 1788 is a human B-lymphoblastoid cell line which produces TNF-β constitutively. If this line is grown in the presence of phorbol myristate acetate (PMA), however, the levels released are increased more than ten-fold (over 500 U/ml). The pro-myelocytic leukaemia HL60 is a human cell line which can be induced to differentiate into monocyte-like cells by the application of phorbol esters. Treatment of these differentiated cells with endotoxin results, after 24 h, in the production and release of TNF-α at levels approaching 400 U/ml. Recombinant prokaryotic and eukaryotic TNF-α and

Table 10.3 Sources of TNF

Cellular source	Stimulant	TNF produced
Macrophages	LPS	TNF-α
Monocytes	LPS	TNF-α
Differentiated HL60	LPS	TNF-α
T-lymphocytes	PHA	TNF-β
	Specific AG	
T-cell hybridomas (some)	Constitutive	TNF-β
CD4$^+$ T-cell clones	AG + Class II +	TNF-β
	APC	
CD8$^+$ T-cell clones	AG on Class I	TNF-β
	matched cells	
RPMI 1788	$\pm$ PMA	TNF-β

Key:
LPS: Lipopolysaccharide
PHA: Phytohaemagglutinin
AG: Antigen
APC: Antigen-presenting cell
PMA: Phorbol myristate acetate

TNF-β are now both available. The use of these is essential in order to establish which activities are due solely to TNF rather than to contaminating molecules. However, the establishment of direct effects is also hampered by the fact that TNF both induces other interleukins such as IL-1 and also synergizes with others, such as IFN-γ.

Assay of TNF

The most common assays for TNF are still bioassays which rely on the cytotoxic or growth inhibitory properties of TNF (Matthews and Neale, 1987).

Cytotoxicity assays.   Both species of TNF can be measured by their ability to cause the lysis of susceptible cell lines *in vitro*. In cytotoxicity assays (Fig. 10.5), target cells are seeded into the wells of microtitre plates at a known cell density. Serially diluted TNF samples are added to the cells and the number of cells remaining after a fixed incubation period can be counted microscopically after fixation and staining. Alternatively, if the cells are stained with a dye then the amount of dye taken up is proportional to the number of cells present and can be measured spectrophotometrically. In other assays, target cells are labelled with

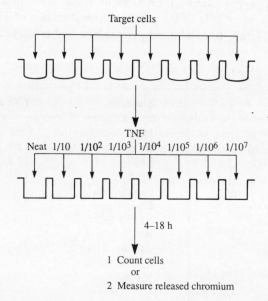

Fig. 10.5 Cytotoxicity assays. Target cells are seeded into plastic multi-well dishes and incubated with serially diluted TNF samples. After a suitable incubation period, the remaining cells are counted. Alternatively, if the targets are pre-labelled with radioactive chromium, the amount of chromium released into the supernatant is a measure of the number of cells killed.

^{51}Cr prior to incubation with TNF. The amount of radiolabel released into the supernatant is used as a measure of cell killing and can be compared both to the amount which is released spontaneously and to the total amount which can be released (usually measured by deliberately lysing the cells with a detergent). The percentage cytotoxicity is calculated by the following formula:

$$\text{Cytotoxicity (\%)} = \frac{\%\,^{51}\text{Cr (test)} - \%\,^{51}\text{Cr (spontaneous)}}{\%\,^{51}\text{Cr (maximum)} - \%\,^{51}\text{Cr (spontaneous)}} \times 100$$

It is very easy to label the cytoplasmic proteins by incubating the target cells with sodium ^{51}Cr for 1–2 h prior to the assay. However the strong tendency of ^{51}Cr-labelled cells to release Cr spontaneously limits the length of the incubation period, ideally to < 18 h and after 24 h the spontaneous release is generally too high to give meaningful results.

Target cells.   Several different target cell lines have been used to assay both species of TNF. One convenient line, which grows well in the laboratory, is the murine tumour L929, an adherent cell line which, when treated with inhibitors of replication, such as actinomycin D or mitomycin C, is particularly susceptible to TNF. In some laboratories, L929 clones have been selected for higher susceptibility to TNF and this produces a corresponding increase in the sensitivity of the assay.

Growth inhibition.   The growth inhibitory effects of TNF can also be measured on human tumour cell lines of which several are widely available. Growth inhibition (as opposed to cytotoxicity) can be measured by looking at DNA synthesis as measured by the uptake of tritiated thymidine into cell cultures. Human TNF can also be assayed by its ability to cause necrosis of human tumours transplanted into athymic mice. Whatever bioassay is used, it may be necessary to establish that the effect is solely attributable to TNF. In such a case, a control using a monoclonal antibody to TNF is essential.

Immunoassay.   With the availability of monoclonal antibodies to TNF, and of pure recombinant TNF, the latest assays for TNF are immunoassays as opposed to bioassays. At least one radioimmunoassay for TNF is now available commercially in a kit form.

Molecular biology of TNF

The first extensive purification of human TNF-α was carried out using the supernatants of endotoxin-induced differentiated HL60 cells (Wang *et al.*, 1985). These monocytes release 300–400 U/ml of TNF when stimulated with endotoxin. Although this level is high in terms of activity, in terms of mass of protein for biochemical characterization, it is very small. For example, purification from 4–8

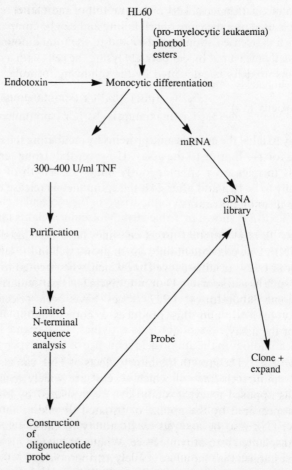

Fig. 10.6 Cloning of TNF-α. The approach to cloning the TNF-α gene is essentially the same as other lymphokines. The producer cell used was the HL60 line which was treated with phorbol esters to induce monocytoid differentiation. When treated with endotoxin these cells release TNF-α which was used both for pure TNF, for sequence analysis, and for mRNA used to construct a cDNA library.

litres of culture supernatant yielded only 10–20 μg of highly purified TNF. Nevertheless, highly purified TNF from HL60 cells was used to determine the N-terminal amino acid sequence and this was then used to synthesize a complementary oligoRNA probe (Fig. 10.6). For gene cloning, mRNA was isolated from induced HL60 cells and used to construct a cDNA library. The library was then screened with the synthetic RNA probe to find the 'right' DNA which was then cloned by insertion into *E. coli* using a plasmid vector.

Human TNF-β, from RPMI 1788 has also been purified biochemically and its amino acid sequence determined. Moreover, the gene for TNF-β has also been

Table 10.4   Molecular characteristics of human TNF-α and TNF-β

Property	TNF-α	TNF-β
Size of mature molecule	17.3 kDa	18.6 kDa
Number of amino acids	157	171
Glycosylation	None	1 N-linked site
Number of disulphide links	1	None
Gene location	6	6
Isoelectric pH	5.3	

cloned and expressed in *E. coli*. A comparison of the molecular characteristics of TNF-α and TNF-β is shown in Table 10.4. Molecular weights larger than those recorded here for recombinant forms have been recorded in the serum of rabbits and mice, the most likely explanation being the presence of dimers and trimers. Although there is only a single gene for TNF-β, the molecule exists in two forms. The major form has 171 amino acids, 23 more than the minor form. Otherwise the two molecules are identical (Gray *et al.*, 1984). Since the activities of TNF-α and TNF-β are identical, the extra amino acids at the N-terminal end of TNF-β are not considered to be essential for its activities. TNF-α and TNF-β have an overall 30% homology in the amino acid sequence of the polypeptide although in two highly conserved regions this figure increases to 50%. Since the two molecules bind to the same cell receptor, these high homology regions may represent the receptor binding sites. The main difference between the two molecules lies in post-translational glycosylation. While human TNF-α is not glycosylated. TNF-β has a single asparagine-linked glycosylation site at position 62. Glycosylation at this site is extensive and increases the molecular mass by nearly 40%. The genes for human TNF-α and TNF-β are closely located on chromosome 6 in humans within the MHC close to the HLA-B region (Fig. 10.7) although each gene is independently regulated. A similar location of TNF genes within the MHC has also been found in other animals and is not without immunological significance. TNF is known to increase the expression of MHC antigens, with consequence for MHC-restricted T-cell activity. It has also been

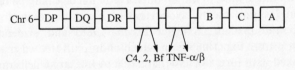

Fig. 10.7   Location of TNF-α/β genes. The genes for both TNF species are located within the MHC of man and mouse. In the HLA region these genes are located 200 kbases centromeric of HLA-B. The TNF-α gene is placed 3' with respect to TNF-β and they are separated by 1.2 kbases.

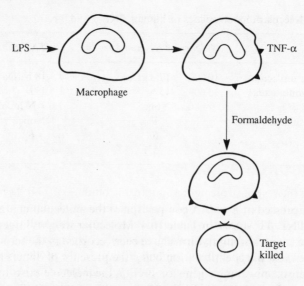

LPS→   Macrophage   → TNF-α

Formaldehyde

Target killed

Fig. 10.8 Membrane-bound TNF-α is toxic. Macrophages were induced to produced TNF-α following treatment with bacterial endotoxin. Some TNF-α remains on the membrane. If the macrophages are fixed in formaldehyde, they are still capable of killing target cells.

suggested that the closeness between the TNF genes and HLA-B in particular, may be in some way related to the development of ankylosing spondylitis, a disease characterized by destruction of intervertebral cartilage, and which is very strongly linked to the HLA-B27 genotype (Carroll *et al.*, 1987).

Transcription of the gene for TNF-α is stimulated in macrophages following endotoxin treatment. The stability of the mRNA is increased if it includes a short sequence of bases upstream from the TNF gene. If this 'stability' sequence is not included, the message is degraded rapidly. The newly synthesized protein contains a long leader sequence of over 70 amino acids, which includes a long hydrophobic region of 20 amino acids in length. The leader sequence is cleaved prior to secretion of the protein but an uncleaved molecule may be retained as a membrane form. It is possible, therefore, that TNF-α exerts some of its effects as a membrane-bound protein (Kriegler *et al.*, 1988) and evidence for this suggestion comes from experiments in which endotoxin-treated macrophages, subsequently fixed with formaldehyde, are able to kill target cells directly (Fig. 10.8). The concept of membrane-bound and soluble TNF is reminiscent of IL-1 which also exists in 'membrane' and 'hormonal' forms. If TNF-β can also exist in a membrane-bound form, it could provide an explanation for short-range killing by CTL.

Table 10.5 TNF receptors on cells

Cells	Number of receptors per cell	Binding affinity
Adipocytes	10 000	3×10^{-9} M
K562 (erythroleukaemia)	3 600	1.6×10^{-10} M
PA-1	1 080	1.6×10^{-10} M

TNF RECEPTORS

The nature of the response brought about by the binding of TNF to receptors on target cells depends on the nature of the target cell itself. Binding of TNF at cell surfaces is followed by receptor-mediated endocytosis although this is probably not a prerequisite for its activity. Indeed, the ability of membrane-bound TNF to destroy cells would support this viewpoint. However, the mode of transmission of the TNF signal after binding is not yet certain although, like most lymphokines studied so far, it is likely to be mediated via protein kinases.

The receptors for TNF on sensitive cells are proteins of approximately 75 kDa. Estimates have been made of the numbers of receptors on target cells by following the binding of radiolabelled TNF at differing concentrations of ligand. These studies have revealed a considerable variation in the number of receptors per cell (Table 10.5). Moreover, the number of receptor per cell is unrelated to the degree of sensitivity of these target cells (Aggarwal *et al.*, 1985). Indeed the largest numbers are sometimes found on relatively insensitive cell lines. The receptors in all cases are of high affinity, with binding affinities in the order of 10^{-10} M.

TNF in therapy

The main area of research into therapeutic effects of TNF has been, as expected, in the field of human tumour therapy. However, the knowledge that TNF also causes septic shock and cachexia, indicates that toxicity of the molecule must be carefully considered. Clinical trials are under way and data are becoming available on both the kinetics of TNF treatment and on the establishment of a maximum tolerated dose. Exogenous TNF has a plasma half-life of 30–60 min and continuous infusion can achieve a steady-state level of 1 U/ml (Warren *et al.*, 1987). Administration of TNF most commonly results in fever, chills, headache, fatigue and hypotension. Relatively few cancer trials have been completed but in Phase I trials to establish toxicity and maximum tolerated doses in cancer patients, occasional tumour regression has been seen, particularly when TNF was injected directly into the tumour. It is fair to say that extensive results of Phase I and II trials with TNF are still awaited and many trials are being conducted worldwide. Combination therapy, in which TNF and IFN-γ are used together, is also being assessed. In some cases, administration of TNF and IFN-γ has resulted in severe pain at the tumour site and it has been suggested that this is due to an effect on the blood vessels in the tumour, perhaps with internal bleeding. Similarly combinations of TNF with other molecules such as IL-2 and IL-1, or even TNF in conjunction with several interleukins, might prove to be the most effective treatment, since it would more closely approximate an '*in vivo*' cytokine cocktail.

Summary

TNF is a generic term given to two structurally related molecules which are the products of the monocyte/macrophage (TNF-α) and the activated lymphocyte (TNF-β). TNF displays potent antitumour activity in animal models and may be useful in treating human tumour patients. TNF also has multiple activities in promoting inflammation, which may account, in part, for the antitumour activity of this molecule. However, the initial euphoria surrounding the discovery of TNF, and the recognition of its tumoricidal properties, has been tempered by the discovery that the same molecule is responsible both for cachexia and septic shock. Any proposals for treating cancer patients with TNF must bear this potential toxicity in mind. On the other hand, the knowledge that TNF is involved in septic shock provides a basis for treating this acute and sometimes fatal illness. Whether the doses which might be effective in treating cancer patients are likely also to stimulate shock needs to be determined. For this reason, Phase I clinical trials have been instigated in several countries in order to establish such parameters; the results of these are eagerly awaited.

References

Aggarwal, B. B., Essalu, T. E. and Hass, P. E. (1985). 'Characterisation of receptors for human tumour necrosis factor and their regulation by interferon-γ', *Nature (London)* **318**, p. 665.

Baldwin, R. W., Embleton, M. J. and Robins, R. A. (1973). 'Cellular and humoral immunity to rat hepatoma-specific antigens correlated with tumour status', *Int. J. Cancer* **11**, p. 1.

Beutler, B., Mahoney, J., Le Trang, N. *et al.* (1985). 'Purification of cachectin, a lipoprotein lipase-suppressing hormone secreted by endotoxin-induced RAW 264.7 cell', *J. Exp. Med.* **161**, p. 984.

Carroll, M. C., Katzman, P., Alicot, E. M. *et al.* (1987). 'Linkage map of the human major histocompatibility complex including the tumor necrosis factor genes', *Proc. Natl Acad. Sci. (USA)* **84**, p. 8535.

Carswell, E. A., Old, L. J., Kassel, R. L. *et al.* (1975). 'An endotoxin-induced serum factor that causes necrosis of tumours', *Proc. Natl Acad. Sci. (USA)* **25**, p. 3666.

Cerami, A. and Beutler, B. (1988). 'The role of cachectin/TNF in endotoxic shock and cachexia', *Immunol. Today* **9**, p. 28.

Dinarello, C. A., Cannon, J. G., Wolff, S. M. *et al.* (1986). 'Tumour necrosis factor (cachectin) is an endogenous pyrogen and induces production of interleukin-1', *J. Exp. Med.* **163**, p. 1433.

Feinman, R., Henriksen-Destefano, D., Tsujimoto, M. and Vilcek, J. (1987). 'Tumor necrosis factor is an important mediator of tumor cell killing by human monocytes', *J. Immunol.* **138**, p. 635.

Gamble, J. R., Harlan, J. M., Klebanoff, S. J. and Vadas, M. A. (1985). 'Stimulation of the adherence of neutrophils to umbilical vein endothelium by human recombinant tumor necrosis factor', *Proc. Natl Acad. Sci. (USA)* **82**, p. 8667.

Grau, G. E., Fajardo, L. F., Piquet, P.-F. *et al.* (1987). 'Tumour necrosis factor (cachectin) as an essential mediator in murine cerebral malaria', *Science* **237**, p. 1210.

Gray, P. W., Aggarwal, B. B., Benton, C. V. *et al.* (1984). 'Cloning and expression of cDNA for human lymphotoxin, a lymphokine with tumour necrosis activity'. *Nature (London)* **312**, p. 721.

Kriegler, M., Perez, C., DeFay, K. *et al.* (1988). 'A novel form of TNF/cachectin is a cell surface cytotoxic membrane protein: ramifications for the complex physiology of TNF', *Cell* **53**, p. 45.

Matthews, N. and Neale, M. L. (1987). 'Cytotoxicity assays for tumour necrosis factor and lymphotoxin', in *Lymphokines and Interferons: A Practical Approach*, Eds Gearing, A. J. M. Morris, A. G. and Clemens, M. J. Oxford, IRL Press.

Matthews, N., Neale, M. L., Jackson, S. K. and Stark, J. M. (1987). 'Tumour cell killing by tumour necrosis factor: inhibition by anaerobic conditions, free radical scavengers and inhibitors of arachidonate metabolism', *Immunology* **62**, p. 153.

Nawroth, P. P., Bank D., Handley, J., *et al.* (1986). Tumor necrosis factor/cachectin interacts with endothelial cell receptors to induce release of interleukin-1. *J. Exp. Med.* **163**, p. 1363.

Tracey, K. J. and Cerami, A. (1988). 'Cachectin/tumour necrosis factor and other cytokines in infectious disease', *Curr. Opin. in Immunol.* **1**, p. 454.

Waage, A., Halstensen, A. and Espevik, T. (1987). 'Association between tumour necrosis factor in serum and fatal outcome in patients with meningococcal disease', *Lancet* **i**, p. 355.

Wang, A. M., Creasey, A. A., Ladner, M. B. *et al.* (1985). 'Molecular cloning of the complementary DNA for human tumour necrosis factor', *Science* **228**, p. 149.

Warren, R. S., Starnes, H. F. Jr, Gabrilove, J. L. *et al.* (1987). 'The acute metabolic effects of tumour necrosis factor administration in humans', *Arch. Surg.* **122**, p. 1396.

Wozebcraift, A. O., Dockrell, H. M., Taverne, J. *et al.* (1984). 'Killing of human malarial parasites by macrophage secretory products', *Infect. Immunol.* **43**, p. 664.

Summary

One of the difficulties in writing a book of this kind, on a topic which is the subject of so much research interest, is the sheer volume of information which is emerging all the time about these molecules. Selection of material, and of the molecules for detailed study, can become a headache. In the previous chapters an attempt has been made to introduce students to the concept of lymphokines and interleukins and to outline the role of some well-known examples which are essential for the correct functioning of an immune response. The number of lymphokines which have been dealt with in this book is by no means exhaustive and several factors which have not yet been assigned interleukin numbers will be cloned and analysed in the near future. Indeed, since starting to write this book (not that long ago) numbers have been assigned to interleukins 4, 5, 6, 7 and, more recently, IL-8. In this short chapter, an attempt will be made, not so much to predict which activities will be named next, but to predict the uses of some of the lymphokines already available. In addition, there are several areas of research which are poised to yield a wealth of essential information which will greatly aid our understanding about the mechanism of action of these molecules.

Nomenclature

The interleukin nomenclature was introduced in order to avoid the confusing situation in which the same molecule was known under many different names. In addition, it avoided the use of a 'function-based' name which could be misleading in terms of the overall activity of that molecule. For example, the name TNF implies almost that the most important activity of this molecule is in inducing necrosis of tumours. Another example might be IFN-γ, which does indeed have a powerful antiviral activity, but which is probably more significant as an immunodulatory substance. However, the application of the interleukin designation is by no means universal and the two molecules just mentioned are a case in point: these molecules are interleukins but without a designation. It does seem to be the ideal time to reconsider interleukin nomenclature, as the multiple activities of these molecules is really beginning to be appreciated. A nomenclature, or an interleukin designation, might be found in which the range of functions could be incorporated, just as, for example, there is a classification of enzymes which incorporates their biochemical activity.

Mechanism of action of lymphokines

The nature of signal transmission across cell membranes generally is only now becoming clearer. Much research is needed to ascertain whether such signal transmission is also important in the mechanism of action of these molecules. A clearer understanding of how they work will have obvious benefits, for example, when a molecule is responsible for a pathological response, blocking the signal transmission might prevent these complications. One prime example is TNF and the development of cachexia, the wasting syndrome which often accompanies cancer and parasitic burden. Monoclonal antibodies to molecules such as TNF, which induce pathological change, might be used to prevent such changes occurring in the first place. However, analysis of the G-proteins involved in signal transmission, and the ways in which these G-proteins might be manipulated, may offer a finer 'tuning' effect.

Overlapping activities of lymphokines

At one time, it was expected that the soluble factors which controlled cell-mediated immunity, or which provided 'help' for antibody production, would be antigen-specific, in much the same way as antibody. On the contrary, these molecules have turned out to be antigen non-specific. The only specificity lies in the stimulation of the specific cells which produce them, and in the target-cell specificity, which is determined by the presence of the correct 'lymphokine' receptor in the cell membrane. The overlapping nature of the biological activities of these molecules has also proved surprising in that several molecules have been found to promote the same activity. For example, both IL-2 and IL-4 can act as T-cell growth factors; both IL-3 and IL-4 can act as mast-cell growth factors. In addition, synergistic effects are increasingly seen to be important. It almost seems irrelevant nowadays to study the effect of a lymphokine *in vitro*, in isolation from the cocktail of lymphokines which are found in the supernatants of activated lymphocytes. This synergy is going to be increasingly important where mixtures of lymphokines are used in treatment of diseases such as AIDS and cancer. Effective treatments may require much more complicated clinical trials in which the efficacy of different combinations of these proteins is evaluated on a scientific basis (as far as it is possible).

Glycosylation

Many of the molecules discussed in this book have considerable amounts of carbohydrate associated with them. This carbohydrate is not essential for the biological activity of these compounds but clearly it must have a role *in vivo*. Many people have the strong feeling that the glycosylation is important since so much cellular 'effort' is invested in it. On the other hand, if unglycosylated molecules are equally effective, specific inhibitors of glycosylation might prove useful in biotechnological terms, conserving that energy which would otherwise go into glycosylation, and possibly increasing the yield of the product.

Lymphokines, interleukins and B-cells

The production of antibody-secreting cells from antigen-stimulated B-lymphocytes is a very complex process, depending, as it does, on the presence of a variety of lymphokines and interleukins. Several of these molecules have been mentioned in previous chapters and yet more are 'on the horizon'. Knowledge of the extent to which T-cell-derived proteins can influence the proliferation and differentiation of B-lymphocytes would be useful for producing human monoclonal antibodies where immunization of a 'volunteer' may be precluded by the hazardous nature of a potential immunogen. Human monoclonal antibodies have advantages over the more usual mouse monoclonals, particularly where they are used for treating patients, when mouse proteins might induce allergic responses.

Lymphokines and the treatment of cancer

The use of lymphokines to treat cancer stems from the observed effects of IFN in inducing inhibition of growth in cultured tumour cells. In addition, both IL-2 and IFN (all classes) were shown to increase the cytotoxicity of NK cells, which spontaneously destroy some cultured tumour cells. Extensive use of IFN in treating cancer of all kinds has generally yielded disappointing results, although the treatment of hairy cell leukaemia with IFN can be accounted a great success. The use of IL-2 in LAK therapy has proved successful, but again with only certain kinds of cancer, such as renal cell carcinoma and malignant melanoma. However, the incidence of severe toxicity associated with this treatment, as well as the logistical problems associated with LAK therapy, suggests that a cautious approach needs to be taken. Clearly, different centres using this therapy worldwide need to evaluate the best ways of overcoming these problems. The proposed use of IL-4 together with IL-2 may prove more effective. If the toxicity is related to other lymphokines induced as a result of IL-2 treatment, administration of specific monoclonal antibodies may be useful. One area of·

cancer treatment in which lymphokines are becoming extremely useful, is the use of haemopoietic growth factors, such as GM-CSF and IL-3, in restoring bone marrow which has been severely depleted, for example, by cytotoxic chemo-therapy. The ability to 'boost' the bone-marrow cells in this way may allow higher doses of drugs to be given, in order to purge the body of remaining cancer cells.

Lymphokines and parasites

Parasitic infections account for millions of deaths worldwide each year. Parasites also cause enormous losses in agricultural terms, particularly in the Third World. The immune response to parasites is only in the last few years being recognized although the role of IgE has been suggested for a number of years. However, the increasing knowledge of the roles and interrelationships between IgE, mast cells, eosinophils, IL-3, IL-4 and IL-5, may provide a means for the treatment of such infections. Moreover, greater knowledge of the role of these molecules in producing an immune response to parasites might be useful in preventing allergic reactions involving IgE, which are very common and, though often trivial, can occasionally be life-threatening.

Lymphokines, interleukins and immunopathology

IL-1, IL-6 and especially TNF, have all been implicated in the development of the muscle wasting which can occur as a result of chronic inflammation, parasitic infection, or the presence of a malignant tumour. Although muscle proteolysis has short-term benefits in an acute inflammatory episode, providing amino acids for proliferating lymphocytes, and for the synthesis of the acute phase proteins, a chronic phase can be extremely debilitating.

Several lymphokines have also been implicated in the development and maintenance of autoimmune disease. In particular, those lymphokines such as IFN-γ and IL-4, which induce the expression of MHC Class II proteins on inappropriate cells, may be a trigger for the initiation of autoimmune reactions. The synovial fluid of involved joints of patients with rheumatoid arthritis is known to contain IL-1, IL-6 and IFN-γ, for example, all of which may promote local inflammatory reactions. IL-6, which supports the growth of myeloma cells *in vitro*, may also be implicated in the development of myeloma *in vivo*.

AIDS

The global incidence of infection with HIV continues to rise exponentially. In some regions of the world the incidence of AIDS, which, it seems, is an almost inevitable consequence of HIV infection, has reached epidemic proportions.

Clearly, even if a vaccine were available tomorrow, the incidence of AIDS will not decrease for many years, and an effective therapy needs to be developed to 'cure' as well as to 'prevent'. One possible treatment, at least to deal with the opportunistic infections of AIDS, is to replace the lymphokines which the patients lose when the helper T-cells are destroyed by the virus. IL-1 and IL-2 have both been used to treat AIDS patients although with limited success. The increasing number of recombinant lymphokines available will make it easier, though no less expensive, to assess the value of combinations of lymphokines in the treatment of these patients.

Index